Helping Children and Young People Who Self-harm

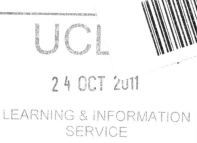

Every year thousands of children and young people attend emergency departments with problems resulting from self-harm. More still come to the attention of Child and Adolescent Mental Health Services teams, school nurses and other community-based services. *Helping Children and Young People Who Self-harm* provides clear and practical guidance for health professionals and other members of the children's workforce who are confronted with this complex and difficult area.

Providing accessible evidence-based advice, this textbook looks at:

- what we mean by self-harm and its prevalence
- the legal background
- what works for young people who self-harm
- what children and young people think about self-harm
- assessment and interventions for self-harm
- prevention of self-harm
- service provision and care pathways.

Essential for all those working with children and young people, this textbook contains a glossary of terms, practical strategies and case studies.

Tim McDougall is a nurse consultant in Child and Adolescent Mental Health Services, Chester.

Marie Armstrong is a nurse consultant in Child and Adolescent Mental Health Services, Nottingham.

Gemma Trainor is a nurse consultant in Child and Adolescent Mental Health Services, Manchester.

Helping Children and Young People Who Self-harm

An introduction to self-harming and suicidal behaviours for health professionals

Tim McDougall, Marie Armstrong and Gemma Trainor

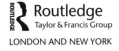
Routledge
Taylor & Francis Group

LONDON AND NEW YORK

6280454

First published 2010
by Routledge
2 Park Square, Milton Park, Abingdon, Oxon, OX14 4RN

Simultaneously published in the USA and Canada
by Routledge
270 Madison Avenue, New York, NY 10016

Routledge is an imprint of the Taylor & Francis Group, an informa business

© 2010 Tim McDougall, Marie Armstrong and Gemma Trainor

Typeset in Garamond by
GreenGate Publishing Services, Tonbridge, Kent

Printed and bound in Great Britain by
CPI Antony Rowe, Chippenham, Wiltshire

British Library Cataloguing in Publication Data
A catalogue record for this book is available from the British Library

Library of Congress Cataloging-in-Publication Data
McDougall, Tim.
Helping children and young people who self harm : an introduction to self-harming
and suicidal behaviours for health professionals / Tim McDougall, Marie Armstrong,
and Gemma Trainor.
p. ; cm.
Includes bibliographical references and index.
1. Self-destructive behavior in children. 2. Self-destructive behavior in adolescence.
3. Parasuicide. 4. Suicidal behavior. I. Armstrong, Marie, 1965- II. Trainor, Gemma.
III. Title.
[DNLM: 1. Self-Injurious Behavior. 2. Adolescent. 3. Child. 4. Suicide. WM 165
M4773h 2010]
RJ506.S39M43 2010
616.85'8200835—dc22   2009052312

ISBN: 978-0-415-49913-2 (hbk)
ISBN: 978-0-415-49914-9 (pbk)
ISBN: 978-0-203-84914-9 (ebk)

Tim: For my wonderful children: Amy, Sam and Jack.

Marie: Thanks to my husband Declan for his support and encouragement, for helping to keep me going when I have deadlines to meet, and to our daughter Maeve for her love and being a fantastic adolescent.

Gemma: Special thanks to George and my beautiful girls, Ciara and Shauna, for being who they are and putting up with the drama.

Contents

Figures

Tables

Contributing authors

Tim McDougall RMN, BSc (Hons), PG Dip, Specialist Practitioner (Mental Health), ENB 603, is part-time nurse consultant (Tier 4 CAMHS) and lead nurse (CAMHS) at the Cheshire & Wirral NHS Foundation Trust. Tim is also part of the North West NHS Children and Families Programme team. Tim has worked in a range of CAMHS settings, including community child mental health teams, adolescent inpatient services and secure adolescent forensic services. With a national profile in CAMHS and, with over 80 book and journal publications, Tim has spoken at national and European conferences about the mental health of children and adolescents. Tim was formerly nurse advisor for CAMHS at the Department of Health in England, and is primarily interested in the strategic development and leadership of CAMHS and nursing. Tim was an expert witness for the National Inquiry into self-harm by young people, and is currently a member of the National Advisory Council for Children's Mental Health and Psychological Wellbeing.

Marie Armstrong is a nurse consultant and clinical lead for the child and adolescent mental health self-harm service in Nottingham. With over 22 years of experience in CAMHS, she has worked in a variety of settings including adolescent inpatient, children's day service, community mental health teams and primary care liaison nursing. Marie has been a nurse consultant since 2000. Her current post involves 50 per cent direct clinical practice as well as leadership and consultancy, teaching, research and service development. Marie has developed and implemented good practice guidelines for the management of young people who self-harm and helped develop the National Institute for Clinical Excellence (NICE) guidelines on self-harm. Marie provides training workshops and speaks at conferences. As well as being trained in child and adolescent mental health nursing, Marie is a qualified and UKCP registered systemic family psychotherapist.

Gemma Trainor, PhD, is a nurse consultant with nearly 30 years of experience working with young people who self-harm. She has spent the last 12 years researching treatments, and was one of the lead investigators in two

xiv   *Contributing authors*

major randomised controlled trials which investigated a group treatment for young people who self-harm. Gemma has published extensively and regularly presents at national and international conferences on promising treatments for self-harm. She was an expert witness for the National Inquiry into self-harm by young people carried out by the Mental Health Foundation and the Camelot Foundation, and is currently a member of the Royal College of Psychiatrists' Steering Group on Self-harm, chaired by Lord Allerdice of Knock.

Foreword

by Professor Keith Hawton

Self-harm in young people is receiving increasing attention from health professionals and the public. This reflects the apparent growing extent of this problem, as reflected in rising numbers of hospital presentations, especially for self-cutting, and the large numbers of adolescents who self-harm but do not come to the attention of clinicians. The increase in self-harm in young people is not just a problem in the UK, but has been documented in several Western countries and in other parts of the world, including some where self-harm has previously been thought to be rare.

Clinicians working in Child and Adolescent Mental Health Services, as well as those in primary care and general hospital settings, need to be fully informed on this topic. This necessitates knowing about the nature and extent of self-harm, what factors contribute to the behaviour, how to assess the young person who is self-harming (including how to relate and talk to youngsters who are often ashamed, desperately unhappy, yet mistrustful of adults), what sources of help are available, and when and how to talk to relatives and carers about the issue. In this book, written by three senior nurses with a wealth of experience of working with youngsters who have self-harmed, Tim McDougall, Marie Armstrong and Gemma Trainor address all these issues in a very practical fashion. Their extensive use of case material, together with quotes and poems, gives the text a very human feel that engages the reader. Importantly, they do not make unrealistic claims, but highlight where we are lacking information, especially in relation to the most effective methods of care. At the same time, their depth of experience is apparent throughout.

This book is primarily aimed at clinicians, who, whether experienced or early in their careers, are equally likely to find this book not only interesting but highly informative. It will also be useful for relatives and carers, and indeed the young people who self-harm. There is a need for more practical and wise guidance on self-harm in children and young people – and this is exactly what this book provides.

Professor Keith Hawton
Director, Centre for Suicide Research, Oxford University Department of Psychiatry,
and *Consultant Psychiatrist, Oxfordshire and Buckinghamshire Mental Health*
NHS Foundation Trust

Foreword

by Dr Cathy Street

For some years now, self-harm among young people has been recognised as a very common problem, however, concern about this issue has become more prominent after the emergence of recent reports highlighting growing rates of depression and general unhappiness among young people, and surveys indicating that just over one-fifth of young people in the UK aged 11–19 years have, at some point, tried to harm themselves.

Understanding the reasons for self-harm is a complex issue, not least because there are varying definitions, but also because much self-harming behaviour is hidden, with young people never seeking help and thus not coming to the attention of health or social care services. As the Mental Health Foundation noted in their introduction to their inquiry, *The truth about self-harm* (Mental Health Foundation 2006), self-harm is a taboo subject, with many young people never revealing that they are self-harming, not even to their closest and most trusted friends.

What we do know, from figures compiled by Oxford University Centre for Suicide Research, is that deliberate self-harm is the reason behind around 170,000 hospital admissions each year of people aged under 35. Therefore, equipping those working in health service settings, in particular Accident and Emergency Departments, to be able to offer appropriate and responsive help, is of critical importance.

Furthermore, from the growing body of research about young people's views of health services, in particular Child and Adolescent Mental Health Services (CAMHS) and adult mental health services, we know a considerable amount about what deters young people from seeking help when struggling with overwhelming worries and difficult feelings – notably, worries about confidentiality and their friends finding out, or about being sent away from home.

The work with young people experiencing mental health difficulties that I have been involved with over the past decade – first at YoungMinds and more recently at Rethink – has also repeatedly highlighted the problem with young people actually not knowing where to go for help. Many also feel that the professionals that they may approach will not understand them, or will not offer advice or help that seems relevant to the difficulties they are experiencing.

This book, with its emphasis on practical advice about how to engage with young people who are self-harming, is based on the authors' many years of experience working directly with young people, and is thus a much-needed and welcome addition to the literature on this challenging topic.

Dr Cathy Street
Young People's Research and Development Lead, Rethink
89 Albert Embankment
London SE1 7TP

Acknowledgements

The authors wish to thank the following people for their help and support in writing this book.

Tim: The team at Chester – Catherine Phillips for her advice about dialectical behaviour therapy; Dr Alison Wood and Dr Andy Cotgrove for their knowledge of the research field; and Carys Jones for her wealth of experience helping young people who struggle with self-harm. Their good practice inspires us all.

Marie: A huge thank you to all the young people who have contributed to this book by sharing their thoughts, ideas and quotes. To all the young people, parents and carers who have helped me to understand more about self-harm; I have felt privileged that they have shared some of their life stories with me. Thanks to Jo, who is doing a great job working as an advocate for young people in CAMHS and for writing a contribution to Chapter 9. Thanks to my team colleagues Wayne, Caroline and Julie for their support and encouragement, and also for their desire to help young people who self-harm by providing the best services possible.

Gemma: I am very grateful to the young people who shared their views and comments and who inform our practice and keep us young. Thanks also to the parents, carers and staff at the McGuiness Unit, Greater Manchester West Mental Health Foundation Trust, who spend substantial periods of time supporting and learning how to respond to the unique and challenging needs of young people in their care.

Note

All the insights, advice and messages provided by young people in this book are real. However, the names of the children and young people concerned and some of their details have been changed. This is to protect their identity and respect their confidentiality.

Abbreviations

A-SPS	Adapted SAD Persons Scale
ACCT	Assessment, Care in Custody and Teamwork
ADHD	Attention deficit hyperactivity disorder
A&E	Accident and Emergency
ASIST	Applied Suicide Intervention Skills Training
ATS	Australian Triage Scale
BDI	Beck Depression Inventory
BHS	Beck Hopelessness Scale
BME	Black and minority ethnic
BSFT	Brief solution-focused therapy
BSS	Beck Scale for Suicide Ideation
CAMHS	Child and Adolescent Mental Health Services
CASE	Child and Adolescent Self-harm in Europe Study
CBT	Cognitive behavioural therapy
CGAS	Children's Global Assessment Scale
CHIPS	ChildLine in Partnership with Schools
COP	Code of Practice
CPA	Care Programme Approach
CRTU	College Research and Training Unit
DBT	Dialectical behaviour therapy
DBT-A	Dialectical behaviour therapy (adolescents)
DGP	Developmental group psychotherapy
DHSS	Department of Health and Social Security
DRO	Differential reinforcement of other behaviour
DSH	Deliberate self-harm
DSM	*Diagnostic and Statistical Manual of Mental Disorders*
ECHR	European Convention on Human Rights
FACE	Functional Analysis of Care Environments
FLASH	Families Learning About Self-Harm
GVAWP	Glasgow Violence Against Women Partnership
GP	General practitioner
HADS	Hospital Anxiety and Depression Rating Scale
HAS	Health Advisory Service
HoNOSCA	Health of the Nation Outcome Scale for Children and Adolescents

HRA	Human Rights Act
HSC	Hopelessness Scale for Children
ICD	*International Classification of Diseases*
LAC	Looked After Children
LASCH	Local Authority Secure Children's Home
LSCB	Local Safeguarding Children Board
MACT	Manual assisted cognitive therapy
MCA	Mental Capacity Act
MHA	Mental Health Act
MST	Multi-systemic therapy
NAWP	Newham Asian Women's Project
NCI/NCISH	National Confidential Inquiry into Suicide and Homicide by People with Mental Illness
NEET	Not in education, employment or training
NHSP	National Healthy Schools Programme
NICE	National Institute for Health and Clinical Excellence
NSF	National Service Framework
NSHN	National Self-Harm Network
NSIB	Non-suicidal self-injurious behaviour
NSPCC	National Society for the Prevention of Cruelty to Children
NSSI	Non-suicidal self-injury
OCD	Obsessive compulsive disorder
ONS	Office for National Statistics
PPI	Public and patient involvement
PSHE	Personal, social and health education
RCP	Royal College of Psychiatrists
RCPCH	Royal College of Paediatrics and Child Health
RCT	Randomised controlled trial
RSM	Repetitive self-mutilation
SAD	Seasonal affective disorder
SDQ	Strengths and Difficulties Questionnaire
SEAL	Social and Emotional Aspects of Learning
SENCO	Special Educational Needs Coordinator
SHIFT	Self-harm Intervention Family Therapy
SIFA	Screening Interview for Adolescents
SNASA	Salford Needs Assessment Schedule for Adolescents
SQUIFA	Screening Questionnaire Interview for Adolescents
SSRI	Selective serotonin reuptake inhibitor
STORM	Skills-based training on risk management
TaMHS	Targeted Mental Health in Schools
TAU	Treatment as usual
UNCRC	United Nations Convention on the Rights of the Child
VAST	Vulnerability Assessment Screening Tool
WHO	World Health Organization
ZPC	Zone of parental control

Introduction

At the time of writing this book a number of important changes are taking place that are adversely affecting children and young people. Britain is struggling through the most serious economic downturn since the Wall St Crash in 1929 and the Great Depression that ensued. The NHS budget is under threat and care and health services for children and young people are vulnerable to cuts. Of course, it is not just young people who are finding things difficult. Their parents and carers are also struggling with the recession. Unemployment is growing, alcohol consumption is increasing and debt levels are rising.

Children and young people are telling and showing us how this is affecting them. Using YouGov, The Princes Trust interviewed over 2,000 young people aged between 16 and 25 across Great Britain. Nearly half said they felt regularly stressed, over a quarter reported that they were often or always down or depressed, and one in ten insisted that life was meaningless (Princes Trust 2009). The most hopeless attitudes were found in the group known by the Government as NEETs (not in education, employment or training). Young people in this group were significantly less happy and lacked confidence in every aspect of their lives. It is well known that suicide rates rise during times of recession, and young people who feel hopeless are at greater risk (Gunnell *et al.* 2009). By the time this book is published, unemployment among the young is expected to be the highest since the 1970s. UK countries have updated their suicide plans to take account of the economic downturn.

Together, these issues should concern each and every one of us. They show all too clearly that many of our nations' children are unhappy and hopeless. A recent report on child well-being published by UNICEF suggested that out of 21 economically advanced nations across the developed world, the UK has the unhappiest children. The growing rates of self-harm among the young bear witness to this. Just as the final touches were being put to the writing of this book, two 'Looked After' girls from Scotland, aged 14 and 15 entered into a suicide pact and, whilst holding hands together, jumped off a bridge to their deaths. Sadly, this was not an isolated incident. Earlier in 2009, Bridgend in South Wales lost several of its young people in a cluster of suicides. The global media frenzy that followed caused distress to the families and friends of those who had died, heightened anxiety of young people in schools and gave unhelpful messages about self-harm and suicide to the general public.

Perhaps Karl Marx was thinking about self-harm when he said that the only antidote to mental suffering is physical pain. These words are often borne out by young people who believe they have no alternative coping strategies but self-harm to cope with stress and adversity and face life's challenges. It would not be a leap of logic to conclude that rates of self-harm and suicide by children and young people are a reflection of the level of emotional pain they are feeling. Despite the extent of this problem, our understanding about the issues and a strategy to address them remain poorly developed.

A recent report from Action for Children, and the New Economics Foundation *Backing the Future*, suggests that the costs to the UK economy of failing to tackle the factors that combine to produce poor outcomes for children and young people may be as much as £4 trillion over two decades (Action for Children and New Economics Foundation 2009). The report goes on to say that providing interventions to prevent psychosocial problems, such as family breakdown, poverty, mental disorder and substance misuse, and intervening early could save the UK economy £486 billion over 20 years. Research on self-harm and suicide consistently shows that the very same potent risk factors contribute to self-harm and suicide. We suggest that this illustrates an important 'invest to save' principle.

As we will see throughout this book, research and evidence from young people and their parents and carers consistently highlights the factors that produce negative outcomes and either cause or maintain their self-harm. In this book we combine evidence-based practice – research studies; with what has become known as practice-based evidence – experiences of helping children and young people who self-harm. Together, the theory and practice insights combine to produce what we consider to be a guide to good practice. We do not claim to have all the answers. Indeed, our joint experience tells us it is not usually solutions that young people are looking for. Rather, it is understanding, compassion and hope when they are feeling misunderstood and hopeless. We do not underestimate the potential for these fundamental ingredients to help bring about positive change in young people's lives.

Chapter 1 of this book explores what self-harm is, and we hope to show that it means different things to different people. We aim to demonstrate that self-harm is socially and culturally bound, and challenge some of the myths and legends about self-harm that have evolved in the public domain and which have contaminated the caring and helping professionals. We suggest that many of these are neither caring nor helpful, and may actually maintain or make a young person's self-harming worse. We urge health professionals to explore their attitudes to self-harm and transform the manner in which they provide health services for children and young people in distress. On behalf of young people, we ask them not to judge, criticise and fail in their duties of care.

Chapter 2 focuses on why self-harm is a common and growing problem among young people. We will see that trauma and abuse, bullying, parental mental disorder and mental health problems are all closely linked to self-harm and suicide. Some young people are depressed, stressed by exam pressure or worried about the shape of their bodies. Others self-harm because they are being abused, or because they are being bullied at school or college. Some young people harm themselves because it is fashionable and a way of fitting in. We do not suggest that any of these factors are causative in themselves. Rather, we propose that it is the combination of stress factors in the context of poorly developed coping strategies and support systems that lead to self-harm and suicidal behaviour among young people.

Perhaps not surprisingly, we suggest that there is no single approach to helping young people who self-harm, and Chapter 3 summarises the small but growing evidence base in relation to efficacy and outcomes. We are mindful that some young people do not want help with their self-harm. We also know that others do want help, but do not know how to access it. However, we also suggest that too many decide not to seek help because what is on offer is poor or out of step with what young people want.

Despite the scale of the problem and a growing body of research and guidance, professionals often struggle to help young people who harm themselves. Of course, there are many examples of skilled and sensitive care which leave young people feeling supported and understood. However, all too often, young people report feeling misunderstood, judged or punished by those who are charged with their care. Many tell us that we pitch help in the wrong direction or chase causal explanations that do not exist. This, young people say, can make their self-harm worse. Chapter 4 draws on the views and stories of young people and discusses what we understand to be unhelpful or even damaging for those who self-harm.

All young people who have self-harmed should have their psychosocial needs assessed. This is to explore psychological, social and motivational factors that have led to self-harm, as well as to evaluate suicidal intent and the young person's level of hopelessness. A thorough and competent assessment should be extensive, dynamic, and rely on several sources of information from young people, parents or carers and teachers or other professionals. For many reasons, the assessment of young people who self-harm is often inadequate.

Chapters 5 and 6 look at how we make sense of a young person's self-harm, consider the risks this may present and then help young people and their parents or carers to manage these risks. To make sense of a young person's self-harm and decide whether or not to intervene, those who seek to help must take account of a range of factors. These relate to the child or young person's age, their wishes and choices, those of their parents or carers and the context in which the self-harm is occurring. Such decisions, if they are to be informed, competent and responsible, are rarely straightforward. Adults have moral, professional and legal obligations to the children and young people in their charge. Decisions about whether to intervene and how to intervene can be helpful or harmful – sometimes with fatal consequences. However, just as it is crucial to assess risk, so, too, it is important to assess protective factors, strengths and resources in the young person, family and wider community network. This is to inform decisions about whether the risks and benefits of professional intervention outweigh the risks of non-intervention.

In Chapter 7 we discuss the available treatments for young people who are suicidal or self-harming. The evidence base for some is extremely limited. However, we suggest from our clinical practice using various individual and group treatments, that it is often the manner in which we engage young people that improves outcomes. That is, it may be less about what we do, and more about the way in which we do it. This hypothesis is currently somewhat untested in research. Feedback from young people and their parents or carers tells us that working in an honest and open way is frequently the key to success. Sharing our views and generating and agreeing collaborative management plans is likely to enable positive outcomes. By contrast, our experience suggests that unilateral decision making and paternalistic interventions are likely to be less successful.

Numerous reports have highlighted that parental involvement is often woefully inadequate, and on occasions parents are excluded from professional care and treatment decisions at the most basic of levels. This is unacceptable and not what any of us would want for our own families. Chapter 8 summarises the views, wishes and needs of parents and carers who support young people who self-harm. We are reminded that having a son or daughter who self-harms or shows suicidal behaviour can be an extremely traumatic experience for parents. Parents report feeling helpless and concerned that they cannot keep their child or young person safe. Such anxieties are often made worse by a lack of information and support from professionals. We suggest that support for parents is often as important as support for children and young people, and better services for parents and carers may contribute to improving long-term positive outcomes. Throughout this book we discuss the impact of stigma on young people who self-harm, as well as on their parents and carers, siblings and friends. Just as stress can build up in a young person who has no appropriate source of support, it can also impact negatively on their social networks. Reducing the stigma associated with self-harm should be a key part of all that we do as health professionals.

The full range of resources and interventions needed by young people who self-harm spans the responsibilities of a range of agencies and services in the public and voluntary sectors. However, care services, including accident and emergency and mental health services, play the greatest role. Chapter 9 describes the service context in which young people who are suicidal or self-harming can access help and support.

Chapter 10 explores what can be done to prevent self-harm and suicide. We suggest that public health strategies that focus on universal interventions to prevent and reduce self-harm by children young people may offset the future burden on paediatric, mental health and social services. However, we propose that this is no easy task and one that requires a comprehensive, integrated effort involving children and young people, families and communities, schools, the media and central government.

It is important that professionals who help children and young people who self-harm are clear about the various legislative frameworks within which they work. This is discussed in Chapter 11. Regardless of their background, professionals should have a working knowledge of human rights legislation, children's rights and mental health law and how these frameworks interact. Despite this, young people often report that they are not involved in decisions, frequently have their privacy, dignity and confidentiality compromised and do not feel that professionals respect them. We suggest that this is unacceptable in twenty-first-century care services.

In summary, we have aimed this book not only at the health sector, but at a wide range of different professionals who together share a responsibility to improve outcomes for children and young people. We hope it will appeal to anyone trying to understand and help those who are struggling with self-harm or feeling suicidal. As well as professionals, we hope to address parents, carers and, of course, young people themselves. Throughout this book we have included their messages about self-harm. These are presented in speech bubbles and serve as reminders to us that adults do not always know best, and that we should always listen carefully to what young people are saying. Finally, we hope we have written a book which will assist health professionals and others to help young people who self-harm change their lives and develop hope and optimism where hopelessness and pessimism have prevailed.

1 What do we mean by self-harm and suicide?

Key points:

- The terms 'self-harm' and 'suicide' are often used interchangeably, frequently causing confusion among professionals as well as children and young people. A number of myths and legends about self-harm have evolved among the general public and caring and helping professionals. Many of these are neither caring nor helpful.
- More often than not, self-harm is not about ending life but is more about regulating emotions, survival and coping with stress. Although self-harm appears on a spectrum with suicide, each has a different pattern and purpose, and interventions to help both have a different foundation and emphasis.
- Phrases such as 'attention seeking' or 'time wasting', or words like 'manipulative' reinforce negative stereotypes about self-harm and can leave young people feeling judged and blamed. Not surprisingly, their experience of health and care services is all too often a negative one. This must be challenged by health professionals.
- Defining self-harm is far from straightforward. Categories often overlap, and the suicidal intent of young people may be changeable or unclear. The term self-harm is therefore often used to describe a young person's behaviour rather than their intent.
- Many people preface the term 'self-harm' with 'deliberate'. However, this is often viewed by young people as derogatory, inferring that the decision to self-harm is thought out and carefully planned. Indeed, self-harm is often impulsive and occurs with little planning or conscious thought. For many reasons, we therefore discourage use of the term deliberate self-harm.
- No single act of self-harm is the same as another, and professionals working with young people need to understand the purpose of self-harm as part of the engagement, risk management and ongoing treatment process. This will evolve as a young person grows, develops and moves towards recovery.
- Trying to define suicidal intent is complex. Research has shown that previous suicidal behaviour in the form of one or more non-fatal suicide

attempts is the most powerful predictor of future suicide. However, the term 'suicide attempt' can be misleading because the majority of acts are not intended to be fatal or even to lead to physical harm.

Introduction

Self-harm and suicidal behaviour, the primary focus of this book, refers to a range of behaviours which are open to interpretation. These are discussed in detail in the following chapters. There is no single, universally agreed definition of self-harm and the term means different things to different people. Self-harm is not limited by age, gender, race, sexual orientation, education, socio-economic status or religion, and how it is recognised and managed varies across the world.

This chapter explores some of the literature defining self-harm and outlines the different terminologies and classifications that are used to describe it. A section on myths and legends is included, and young people's thoughts on the meaning of self-harm are explored. The concluding part of this chapter summarises the debate on some of the factors which may determine whether self-harm is self-destructive or suicidal.

It is not the aim of this chapter to arrive at a definitive term for self-harm. This is because no single definition encompasses all situations. It is hoped that by describing the range of issues to consider when evaluating self-harm, professionals can develop strategies to meet the differing and often complex needs of young people who are suicidal or self-harming.

What is and what is not self-harm?

While the term self-harm may at first seem self-explanatory, a universally accepted definition of the phenomenon is not easy to find. For example, it is only recently that the *Oxford English Dictionary* has included a definition for self-harm: 'Deliberate injury to oneself, typically as a manifestation of a psychological or psychiatric disorder'. Different professionals and the organisations within which they work use a range of words and terms to describe self-harm. Their definitions can vary from short explanations such as the one offered by the National Institute for Clinical Excellence (NICE) Guidelines on Self-harm (NICE 2004a: 16): 'Self poisoning or injury, irrespective of the apparent purpose of the act', to longer and more specific definitions, such as one used in 1989 by the World Health Organization (Platt *et al.* 1992: 92):

> An act with a non-fatal outcome in which an individual deliberately initiates a non-habitual behaviour that, without intervention from others will cause self-harm, or deliberately ingests a substance in excess of the prescribed or generally recognised therapeutic dosage and which is aimed at realising changes which the subject desired via the actual or expected physical consequences.

The working definition used by the International CASE (Child and Adolescent Self-harm in Europe) study group (Madge *et al.* 2008) is an act with a non-fatal outcome in which an individual deliberately did one or more of the following:

- initiated behaviour (e.g. self-cutting or jumping from a height), which they intended to cause self-harm;
- ingested a substance in excess of the prescribed or generally recognised therapeutic dose;
- ingested a recreational or illicit drug that was an act that the person regarded as self-harm;
- ingested a non-ingestible substance or object.

The National Inquiry into self-harm among young people

The National Inquiry into self-harm, *Truth Hurts*, which is discussed throughout this book, considers young people's views about self-harm (Mental Health Foundation and Camelot Foundation 2006). The Inquiry describes self-harm as a wide range of things that people do to themselves in a deliberate and usually hidden way, which are damaging. This includes overdoses and self-mutilation, burning, scalding, banging heads and other body parts against walls, hair pulling, biting, and swallowing or inserting objects.

The National Inquiry chose not look at eating disorders, drug and alcohol misuse, risk-taking behaviours, such as unsafe sex or dangerous driving, in their description of self-harm. They considered that eating disorder behaviours and drug abuse are viewed as self-destructive acts, but focused specifically on self-injury and suicidal behaviour (Mental Health Foundation and Camelot Foundation 2006).

Given the range and variety of definitions and descriptions of self-harm, it is not the intention of this chapter to identify a definition that fits all circumstances. Rather, the objective is to examine various constructs of self-harm to arrive at a more complete understanding of the characteristics, features and motivational factors that combine to produce self-harm.

Apart from the many features of self-harm, the diverse nature, orientation and objectives of organisations working with self-harming individuals requires each to have a slightly different emphasis in their definition. So, even if a unified definition were possible, some would argue that it may not be necessary. It is also important to state that a lot of the professional and academic literature which attempts to make sense of self-harm is based on the experiences of adults, and may not be directly applicable to children and young people.

What is not generally regarded as self-harm?

We all do things that may not be good for us and at times may even be harmful. Overeating, smoking and binge drinking are just a few of the things that are certainly not good for us in the long term, but the physical effects may not be immediate. Practices such as tattooing or piercings are increasingly viewed as acceptable and are often culturally sanctioned. In some cultures, body modifications are symbolic and have religious significance endorsed by a prevailing culture; they each have meaning for the individual, and it is this meaning that needs to be understood by professionals.

Although there is general agreement that they are potentially damaging, risk-taking behaviour, such as excessive drug and alcohol misuse, unsafe sex and over-exercise are not usually regarded as self-harming. Accidental overdoses of alcohol and recreational drugs are rarely seen as specific self-harming behaviours since alcohol and drugs are an inherent part of normal adolescence for many young people (Pryjmachuk and Trainor in press). However, there is evidence that substance misuse among young people is increasing, and both drug and alcohol misuse is related to self-harm and suicide by young people (Rossow *et al.* 2009; Martunnen *et al.* 1991).

Body modification

Body modification, or body alteration, can be defined as the deliberate altering of one's body for non-medical reasons. It includes body piercing, tattooing and implants. Whilst some have suggested that so-called body modification, such as piercing and tattooing, is no different to self-harm through cutting, the distinctions appear to outweigh the similarities. Writing in the 1980s, Walsh and Rosen created four categories in an attempt to differentiate self-harm and address the issue of what might be now regarded as socially acceptable self-harm (see Table 1.1).

Table 1.1 Classification of self-harm (adapted from Walsh and Rosen 1988)

Classification	Examples of behaviour	Degree of physical damage	Psychological state	Social acceptability
I	Ear piercing, nail biting, small tattoos, cosmetic surgery	Superficial to mild	Benign	Mostly acceptable
II	Piercings, machete scars, ritualistic clan scarring, sailor and gang tattoos	Mild to moderate	Benign to agitated	Accepted within subcultures
III	Wrist or body cutting, self-inflicted cigarette burning and tattoos, wound excoriation	Mild to moderate	Psychic crisis	Accepted by some subcultures but not by the general population
IV	Self-castration, eye removal, self-amputation	Severe	Psychotic decompensation	Unacceptable

Reliable psychosocial data about the relationship between body piercing and tattooing are few and controversial (Stirn and Hinz 2008). Tattoos and body piercing have been cultural rituals and initiations for thousands of years both in primitive tribes and highly developed societies.

Self-harm, by comparison, is a largely modern phenomenon. However, what was once considered a social rite or tradition in ancient societies has, for many young people today, become an act of rebellion, often met with disapproval and displeasure from adults. Indeed, body piercing and professional tattoos may seem to meet some of the elements of self-harm in that they are acquired intentionally and involve bodily harm. However, most people consider tattoos and body piercings to be a way of enhancing their appearance or making a statement. Body modifications of this type can be symbolic and endorsed by social groups.

Eating disorders

Other forms of indirect self-harm include eating disorder behaviour, such as anorexia or bulimia nervosa, binge eating and obesity. Some eating disorders are associated with a greater risk of death, suicide and self-harm than others (NICE 2004b). Bulimia nervosa, in particular, is closely linked to self-harm, and young people are at risk both as a result of the disorder and its complications. However, many view risk taking and the harm generated from behaviours associated with eating disorders as separate, requiring a different type of intervention (Favaro and Santonastaso 2000).

Indirect self-harm, in essence, refers to behaviour in which the damage is accumulative as opposed to immediate. Walsh (2006) reviewed a spectrum of self-destructive behaviours and these are summarised in Table 1.2.

Table 1.2 Examples of direct and indirect self-harm (adapted from Walsh 2006)

Direct self-harm	*Indirect self-harm*
• Suicide attempts (e.g. serious overdose, hanging, jumping off a building, use of a gun). • Major self-injury (e.g. eye removal, self amputation. • Atypical self-injury (mutilation of the face, eyes, genitals, breasts). • Common forms of self-injury (e.g. wrist, arm and leg cutting, self burning).	• Substance abuse (e.g. alcohol, drugs). • Eating disorder behaviour (e.g. anorexia nervosa, bulimia, obesity, use of laxatives). • Physical risk taking (walking on a roof or running across the road in high speed traffic). • Situational risk taking (e.g. getting into a car with strangers, walking alone in a dangerous area). • Sexual risk taking (e.g. having unprotected sex with strangers). • Unauthorised discontinuance of psychotropic medications (e.g. misuse or abuse of prescribed medications).

Deliberate self-harm

Health professionals often use the term 'deliberate self-harm' (DSH). This may be misleading since the term 'deliberate' implies premeditation and wilfulness (Pembroke 1994). Indeed, self-harm is atypical, often spontaneous and not obviously preceded by awareness, conscious thought or deliberation. The phrase deliberate self-harm can be used pejoratively and may lead to value judgements being made about the individuals involved (Anderson *et al.* 2004). Some researchers have also referred to a 'deliberate self-harm syndrome', characterised by onset during adolescence, multiple recurrent episodes, low lethality, harm deliberately inflicted on the body, and extension of the behaviour over many years (Pattison and Kahan 1983).

Comparing descriptions

Before going any further, it may be helpful to look at some of the descriptions used by key organisations, professional groups and recognised self-help networks. Whilst there are undoubtedly common themes in what each constitutes as self-harm, the words and phrases used are not always used consistently, and at times may be contradictory.

There are some interesting differences, particularly those related to potential causes, which are important when we come to discuss strategies for intervention. Ensuring successful strategies are adopted when responding to self-harm requires careful investigation and sound understanding of the expression of self-harming behaviour by professionals. As we will see throughout this book, this can only be achieved in consultation with the young people themselves and their parents or carers, and what works for one young person may not necessarily be effective for another.

Therefore, making sense of the words each young person uses to describe their self-harm is crucially important, and sets the context for any subsequent helping intervention if this is required. Table 1.3 compares different brief descriptions used by some key organisations and information portals.

The terms self-injury and self-harm are often used interchangeably. It is easy to see how confusion may develop when describing, discussing and evaluating self-harming behaviours. Considering both fatal and non-fatal acts is part of the *Health for All* targets of the World Health Organization (WHO 2009). Therefore, some would argue that obtaining a consistent formulation is much needed.

An historical perspective

The concept of self-harm has been evolving in the research literature since the early twentieth century. Described using many different words and phrases, Emerson (1913) considered self-cutting to be a symbolic substitution for masturbation.

Table 1.3 Examples of how self-harm is described by different groups

Source	Descriptions
Royal College of Psychiatrists	Self-harm happens when someone hurts or harms themselves. It can feel to other people that these things are done coolly and deliberately – almost cynically. But someone who self-harms will usually do it in a state of high emotion, distress and unbearable inner turmoil. Some people plan it in advance, others do it suddenly. Some people self-harm only once or twice but others do it regularly. It can become almost like an addiction.
NHS Direct	Self-injury or self-harm is when somebody damages or injures their body on purpose. Self-injury is a way of expressing deep emotional feelings or problems that build up inside.
Mental Health Foundation	Self-harm describes a wide range of things that people do to themselves in a deliberate and usually hidden way. In the vast majority of cases self-harm remains a secretive behaviour that can go on for a long time without being discovered.
TheSite.org	People who self-harm deliberately injure themselves mostly as a way of coping with painful and difficult feelings. They are not usually trying to commit suicide but are thought to be more likely to eventually do so.
Selfharm.org.uk	Self-harm is when someone deliberately hurts or injures him or herself. Some young people self-harm on a regular basis while others do it just once or a few times. For some people it is part of coping with a specific problem and they stop once the problem is resolved. Other people self-harm for years whenever certain kinds of pressures or feelings arise.
MIND	Self-harm is a way of expressing very deep distress. Often people don't know why they self-harm. It is a means of communicating what can't be put into words or even into thoughts and has been described as an inner scream. Afterwards people feel better able to cope with life again for a while.
CHILDLINE	Self-harm is when people set out to harm themselves deliberately, sometimes in a secret way. Self-harm can include cutting, burning, bruising or poisoning but does not usually mean that someone wants to commit suicide. Self-harm help and support is available from us anytime you feel like hurting yourself.
Helpguide.org	Self-injury, self-inflicted violence, self-injurious behaviour or self-mutilation is defined as a deliberate, intentional injury to one's own body that causes tissue damage or leaves marks for more than a few minutes which is done to cope with an overwhelming or distressing situation.
NICE (2004a)	Intentional self-poisoning or injury irrespective of the apparent purpose of the act.

In the 1930s, Karl Menninger classified what he called 'self- mutilation' into several categories. These were:

1   *Neurotic* – nail biters, pickers, extreme hair removal and unnecessary cosmetic surgery.
2   *Religious* – self-flagellants and others.
3   *Puberty rites* – hymen removal, circumcision or clitoral alteration.
4   *Psychotic* – eye or ear removal, genital self-mutilation and extreme amputation.
5   *Organic brain diseases* – which allow repetitive head banging, hand biting, finger fracturing or eye removal.
6   *Conventional* – nail clipping, trimming or hair and shaving beards.

In some ways, Menninger was ahead of his time when he asserted that when supporting people who self-harm, attitudes are more important than facts (Menninger 1938).

Terminology has been refined somewhat since the twentieth century, but only on a gradual basis. Pao (1969) made a distinction between low lethality, or 'delicate' self-harm, and what he called high lethality or 'coarse' self-harm. Writing in the *British Journal of Medical Psychology*, he proposed that so-called 'delicate cutters' were young and generally had a diagnosis of borderline personality disorder. By contrast, so-called 'coarse cutters' were older and generally thought to be psychotic.

In the 1960s, researchers proposed that suicidal intent should no longer be regarded as essential in self-harm nomenclature. It became increasingly recognised that many people who attempted suicide performed their acts in the belief that they were comparatively safe, aware even in the heat of the moment that they would survive (Kessel and Grossman 1961).

Consequently, in some circles, the term 'attempted suicide' has gradually been replaced by 'deliberate self poisoning' and 'deliberate self-harm'. The terms were chosen to differentiate between accidental and non-accidental events. By the end of the 1960s these terms were widely used by psychiatrists and other professionals. It was not until the 1970s that the paradigm of self-harm shifted away from psychosexual explanations, such as those proposed by Emerson.

By the early 1980s, other terms such as 'parasuicide' had been introduced. This term excludes the question of whether death was a desired outcome. Around the same time, other terms such as 'self-mutilation' evolved, but later this was viewed as being too extreme, implying radical cutting or maiming which would account for only a minority of episodes. More recently, the term 'self-injury' has been adopted and is now more commonly used in this field (Simeon and Favazza 2007).

It is also no longer appropriate to describe someone as committing suicide, since suicide is no longer regarded as a crime. One of the reasons deliberation continues about self-harm and suicide is because no one term absolutely or accurately defines all acts. Acknowledging the complexities involved, the term 'self-harm' is used to describe to a range of behaviours that are discussed throughout this book.

Deconstructing self-harm

In attempting to understand and describe self-harm, various researchers have sought to deconstruct the concept. Kahan and Pattison (1984) identified three components of self-harming acts involving directedness, lethality and repetition. Table 1.4 summarises the components of self-harming acts, giving examples involving each combination of the following factors.

Directedness

This refers to how intentional the behaviour is, if an act is completed in a brief period of time and whether the person had full awareness of its harmful effects. It is considered direct if there was a conscious intention to produce these effects. Otherwise it is viewed as an indirect method of self-harm.

Lethality

This refers to the likelihood of death resulting from the act. Death is usually the intent of the person undertaking the act either immediately or in the near future. However, the need to establish whether a young person wishes to die and what they understand by death is crucially important. Rather than the professional's opinion, it is the young person's perception of, or belief in, potential lethality that matters.

Repetition

This refers to whether or not the act is done more than once, or frequently over a period of time, in other words repeatedly. Young people who self-harm frequently require multiple interventions. However, it is important that health professionals do not become complacent and fail to assess the self-harm and associated risks accurately.

Table 1.4 Components of self-harming acts (adapted from Kahan and Pattison 1984)

Repetitive in nature	Direct behaviours		Indirect behaviours	
	High lethality	Low lethality	High lethality	Low lethality
Yes	Taking small doses of poison over time	Self-injury cutting. Burning, bruising, etc.	Type 1 diabetic not injecting insulin	Smoking, alcoholism
No	Gunshot wound to head	Major self-mutilation	Terminal cancer patient refusing chemotherapy	Walking around town alone at night

Therefore, it is important to consider each episode of self-harm individually. The challenge is to assess risk and help manage the crisis without acting in ways which minimalise the self-harming behaviour of the young person and invalidate their experience.

Non-suicidal self-injury

Non-suicidal self-injury (NSSI) is one of the more recent descriptions used to explain self-harm. NSSI is defined as the direct, deliberate destruction of one's own body tissue in the absence of intent to die (Nock 2009; Nock *et al.* 2009). These features distinguish it from behaviour involving harmful consequences which are not unintended (e.g. lung cancer from smoking) and from suicidal behaviour.

Nock states that NSSI is conceptualised as a harmful behaviour that can serve several intrapersonal (e.g. affect regulation) and interpersonal (e.g. help seeking) functions. NSSI most often involves cutting oneself with a knife, razor or other sharp implement. Typically, it begins in adolescence and among people with a wide range of psychiatric disorders. However, as we will see in Chapter 2, the majority of young people who self-harm do not have a mental disorder.

Nock's thesis primarily focuses on a theoretical model of the development and maintenance of NSSI rather than seeing it as a symptom of a psychiatric disorder. He views it as a function of a means of regulating emotion and explains that social modelling may be why people choose to use NSSI. Other people may use non-injurious ways to regulate their emotions, such as alcohol use, exercise or by verbally communicating with others. In contrast, those who engage in NSSI may have observed the behaviour being used by others or have experienced invalidating environments. This is discussed in more depth later.

Nock stresses that NSSI is not symptomatic of any mental disorder. Instead, he proposes that it may be used to provide an intense signal which, because of its intensity, is more likely to be recognised by others. He views it as quick and easily accessible which, like alcohol, may be attractive to adolescents (Nock 2009).

Non-suicidal self-injurious behaviour

Another term which has been introduced in recent years is non-suicidal self-injurious behaviour (NSIB). This is defined as intentionally injuring oneself in a manner that results in damage to body tissue, and again it is characterised as being without any conscious suicidal intent. NSIB is viewed as falling into the larger spectrum of adolescent suicidal behaviours. However, this may be misleading because, by definition, it is said to involve no suicidal intent. In this analysis, because intent is changeable and not consistent, NSIB falls into the category of suicidality.

Other descriptive terms

The following terms are found in the research literature and are sometimes used to describe self-harm:

- self-injury
- deliberate injury
- self-inflicted injury
- self-inflicted violence
- self-injurious behaviour
- self-mutilation
- intentional injury to one's body
- parasuicide
- attempted suicide.

A good way to understand the range of terms used to describe self-harm would be to perceive them as part of a continuum. This has suicidal ideation at one end, moving through to non-fatal injury to completed suicide at the other end. Some young people only ever experience suicidal ideation. These thoughts may be fleeting and never lead to self-harm. Others may act on their thoughts and self-harm by cutting or burning. Their self-harm may be of low lethality and have no association with suicidal intent. Young people may also follow this continuum to attempt suicide, for example, by overdosing or hanging. In this instance, the intent would be greater and the lethality higher.

Schreidman (1993) differentiates between the intent of a suicidal person opposed to the intent of a self-injuring person. He suggests that the motivation for a suicidal person is to terminate consciousness, whereas self-injury is more to modify consciousness by relieving emotions. What is known from outcomes research is that young people who attempt suicide are much more likely to go on to complete suicide than those in the general population (Social Care Institute for Excellence 2005).

A Swedish study found that four per cent of adolescents had killed themselves when the sample was followed up 10–20 years later (Otto 1972). Thus, whilst the majority of self-harming episodes are not about intent to die, a minority of young people are at risk of completion. Therefore, prevention and early intervention for young people at risk of suicide is imperative. This is discussed further in Chapter 10.

It is helpful for professionals to consider that every act of self-harm is a unique expression to each individual young person. Clinicians working with young people need to understand the intentions of a young person who self-harms as part of the engagement, risk management and ongoing treatment process. Because of the confusion with terminology we have heard about, it is also important to encourage the young person to describe the behaviour in their own words. Avoiding terms such as suicide attempt or parasuicide may enable the young person to speak freely, thus preventing misdiagnosis of the key problems the young person may be facing.

Concepts of self-harm and suicide

Professionals and the wider public often confuse self-harm with suicide attempts. However, many argue that self-harm can be regarded as the opposite of suicide, as it is often a way of coping with life rather than ending it. As with self-harm, academics and clinicians have grappled with definitions of suicide. Diekstra refers to suicide as death that directly or indirectly results from an act that the dead person believed would result in this end (Diekstra 1995).

Similarly, parasuicide, as originally proposed by Kreitman (1977), refers to behaviours involving self-harm where there is little or no intent to kill oneself (Kerfoot 2000). In addition, suicidal thoughts may exist on their own and are not necessarily associated with suicidal behaviour (National Collaborating Centre for Women's and Children's Health 2009). Despite the distinctions, around one third of adolescents who kill themselves have a history of self-harm (Martunnen *et al.* 1991).

There is general agreement that self-harm exists without necessarily intending to end one's life, whereas in definitions of suicide there needs to be a deliberate and direct intent to end life. Currently, WHO have chosen to use the term 'suicide attempt' any time a self-harming individual does not die, regardless of suicide intent (Bille-Brahe *et al.* 2004).

Of course, self-harm is a common precursor to suicide, and people who self-harm may kill themselves by accident. Furthermore, a young person can be self-harming and suicidal at the same time, but the two terms do not mean the same thing. Whilst it is generally considered that suicidal intent is not a part of self-harming behaviour, self-harming behaviour may be potentially life-threatening. However, to think of all young people who self-harm as suicidal is, in the majority of cases, inaccurate (Schmidtke *et al.* 1996; Suyemoto 1998). Consequently, the term self-harm is increasingly used to denote any non-fatal acts, irrespective of the intention.

Trying to define and specify suicidal intent is extremely complex. Numerous studies have shown that previous suicidal behaviour in the form of one or more non-fatal suicide attempts is the most powerful predictor of future suicide (Egmond and van Diekstra 1989). However, the term suicide attempt (parasuicide) can be misleading because the majority of acts are not intended to be fatal or even to lead to physical harm. In their book focusing on suicide in adolescence, Diekstra and Hawton (1987) suggest that different motives can be subsumed under three categories (see Table 1.5).

Diekstra and Hawton propose that most expressions of suicide by adolescents are a combination of interruption and appeal. However, other factors need to be taken into consideration when evaluating self-harming behaviour in order to convey a more comprehensive understanding of what self-harm means for each young person.

Table 1.5 Motives for suicide and self-harm (adapted from Diekstra and Hawton 1987)

* *Cessation* (stopping consciousness, death).
* *Interruption* (interrupting conscious experience briefly, to sleep, not to feel anything temporarily).
* *Appeal* (to affect behaviour in others or elicit care response).

What does self-harm actually involve?

In reaching an understanding about self-harm as opposed to a specific definition, one should explore what is viewed as features of the behaviour. Table 1.6 shows a range of self-harming behaviours which are described on several relevant and influential websites. These organisations between themselves have identified five or six key behaviours, and in doing so have identified 23 different types of behaviour. All descriptions have identified 'cutting' as a key behaviour, with 'burning', 'overdosing', 'skin scratching' and 'hair pulling' featuring prominently. As mentioned previously, only one organisation (MIND) has cited 'risk-taking behaviour' and 'eating disorders' as some of its key defining features of self-harm.

Table 1.6 illustrates the wide range of behaviours which may be considered to fall within the range of what constitutes self-harm, and of course the list is not exhaustive.

Some features and characteristics of self-harm

Some high quality evidence describing the features of self-harm among adolescents is available from a cross-sectional survey of over 6,000 pupils (aged 15–16) from 41 schools in England using self-reported information conducted by Hawton and colleagues (2002). Self-harm in the previous year was reported by 509 (8.6 per cent) pupils, with 179 saying they had wanted to die. Self-harm within the previous year was over three times more common in females than it was in males (11.2 per cent versus 3.2 per cent).

The prevalence for self-harm of 8.6 per cent (past year) and 13.2 per cent (lifetime) are similar to those from the largest equivalent study in the United States (Centers for Disease Control 1990). Within the 509 cases reported by Hawton *et al.*, the two main methods used for self-harm were cutting (257 cases: 64.6 per cent) and poisoning (122 cases: 30.7 per cent). The researchers highlighted a number of other themes in this study. They reported that self-harm was:

* less common in Asian than white females
* more common in females living with one parent
* more common in pupils who had been bullied
* incrementally higher for young people who smoked cigarettes or used alcohol or drugs
* strongly associated with physical and sexual abuse in both sexes
* associated with depression, anxiety, impulsivity and self-esteem in both sexes.

Table 1.6 Key behaviours highlighted by organisations describing self-harm

Behaviour	Organisation								
	HWB	NI	SH	MIND	RCP	MHF	CL	HG	NICE (2004a)
Cutting	✓	✓	✓	✓	✓	✓	✓	✓	✓
Burning/brandishing	✓	✓		✓	✓	✓	✓	✓	✓
Overdose	✓	✓		✓	✓	✓			✓
Skin picking/scratching	✓	✓	✓			✓	✓	✓	
Bruising	✓					✓			
Tearing out hair	✓	✓	✓			✓	✓	✓	
Throwing oneself against something		✓		✓	✓				
Pulling out eyelashes			✓						
Inhaling substances			✓						
Swallowing objects	✓			✓		✓			
Taking unnecessary risks				✓					
Eating disorders				✓					
Alcohol/drug addiction				✓					
Neglecting own emotional/physical needs				✓					
Banging head		✓			✓				
Punching themselves		✓			✓				
Inserting objects					✓				
Scalding		✓				✓			
Breaking bones		✓				✓	✓	✓	
Hitting								✓	
Multiple piercing								✓	
Drinking harmful chemicals		✓						✓	
Asphyxiation									✓

Sources
HWB   Health and Well Being website
NI   National Inquiry into self-harm among young people
SH   Self-harm website
MIND   MIND (mental health charity) website
RCP   Royal College of Psychiatrists website
MHF   Mental Health Foundation website
CL   ChildLine website
HG   Helpguide website
NICE   National Institute of Clinical Excellence website

Having said this, self-harming young people form an extremely heterogeneous group and self-harm affects young people from many different backgrounds and creeds. Different methods of self-harming can denote different expressions. Some young people cut when they are anxious and burn themselves when they are angry. Some use multiple methods and the type of self-harm they engage in may be dictated by availability or means and the circumstances they are in.

In general, self-harm occurs much more often than suicide attempts. People who cut often do so frequently, and their self-harming behaviour may last for many years. People who are actively suicidal often report feeling no better after an attempt, whereas young people who cut may do so in order to feel better, calmer and less emotionally distressed.

Repetition of self-harm

It is important to understand the developmental course of self-harm. Some young people may self-harm only once in their lifetime and rarely require ongoing therapeutic interventions, whereas others continue to self-harm and may require ongoing help. No intervention is known which can stop self-harm altogether, but there are therapies that can successfully reduce the amount a young person self-harms. Young people can also be reluctant to say they self-harm altogether (Social Care Institute for Excellence 2005).

Perhaps not surprisingly, Spirito *et al.* (1989) suggested that many adolescents who self-harm continue to experience difficulties after their first attempt. Repetition of self-harming behaviour often, but not always, indicates that the young person has a higher degree of disturbance and greater psychosocial needs than those who harm only once. Kreitmen and Casey (1988) noted that those who repeat are often high consumers of health service resources. Follow-up studies of adolescents have suggested that approximately one in ten will make a further attempt during the first year (Hawton *et al.* 1996; Hawton *et al.* 2003).

Young people who repeatedly self-harm, compared to non-repeaters, are more likely to have ongoing stresses, difficulties in school, and more serious suicidal intent (Gispart *et al.* 1987; Social Care Institute for Excellence 2005). Pfeffer and colleagues (1993) carried out a six to eight year comparative study of 100 child and adolescent inpatients in New York. The strongest risk factor for repeat suicide attempt was found to be the presence of a mood disorder. The researchers concluded that repetition was often linked to episodes of depression (Pfeffer *et al.* 1993).

A number of narratives have suggested that people who self-harm may go on to become suicidal or attempt suicide by a different method (Lefeure 1996; Spandler 2001). For example, a young person who regularly cuts him or her self may attempt suicide by a different method, such as hanging or overdosing (Bywaters and Rolfe 2002). It is important, therefore, to comprehensively evaluate self-harming behaviours and risks as part of the assessment process. This is discussed further in Chapters 5 and 6.

Formal classification of self-harm

Self-harm is not classified as a mental disorder. NICE have published guide-lines on the short-term physical and psychological management of self-harm in primary and secondary care (NICE 2004a). The evidence-based practice and good practice points from these guidelines are discussed further in Chapter 3 and are referenced throughout this book. NICE suggest that self-harm is not an illness, but is more or less dangerous behaviour that should alert us to an underlying problem, difficulty or disorder (NICE 2004a). The guidance makes distinctions about self-harm depending on the age of the person involved.

The causes or reasons for self-harm are many and varied, and this will be explored more fully in other chapters. The NICE guidelines suggest that treatment should not be based solely on the service user's history, nor that any assumptions should be made based on this history. Instead, each epi-sode of self-harm should be regarded as a separate and individual event with insular causes. Whilst self-harm is often present in those with mental health difficulties, the majority of young people who self-harm do so as a result of their social or environmental circumstances. Self-harm directly associated with psychiatric causes is much less common.

The two main classification systems for mental disorder are the International *Classification of Diseases* (ICD) and the *Diagnostic and Statistical Manual of Mental Disorders* (DSM). However, neither provides diagnostic criteria for self-harm.

International Classification of Diseases (ICD-10)

The *ICD-10* is a multi-axial classification framework for diagnosing a range of mental disorders (WHO 1993) and is the preferred system used in the UK and most European countries. Axis four of the *ICD-10* contains 24 clas-sifications of self-harm which are based on the agent responsible for the harm rather than the nature or reason for self-harm itself.

Codes are used to classify self-harm involving pharmaceuticals, drugs, alco-hol, gases and pesticides; self-harm by physical means, such as drowning, jumping from high buildings, hot objects; and self-harm inflicted by moving objects, such as cars or trains (see Table 1.7).

Diagnostic and Statistical Manual of Mental Disorders

The *Diagnostic and Statistical Manual of Mental Disorders* (DSM-IV) (American Psychiatric Association 1994) is a handbook for mental health professionals which includes standardised diagnostic criteria for a range of mental disor-ders, and is used across North America. The closest the *DSM-IV* comes to a self-harm scale is in the overdose section of Axis III where 24 subcategories of potential drug poisons are listed.

Table 1.7 ICD-10 classification of self-harm

Code	Descriptor
X60	Intentional self poisoning by and exposure to nonopiod analgesics, antipyretics and antirheumatics
X61	Intentional self poisoning by and exposure to antiepileptic, sedative-hypnotic, antiparkinsonism and psychotropic drugs, not elsewhere classified
X62	Intentional self poisoning by and exposure to narcotics and psychodysleptics (hallucinogens), not elsewhere classified
X63	Intentional self poisoning by and exposure to other drugs acting on the autonomic nervous system
X64	Intentional self poisoning by and exposure to other and unspecified drugs and biological substances
X65	Intentional self poisoning by and exposure to alcohol
X66	Intentional self poisoning by and exposure to organic solvents and halogenated hydrocarbons and their vapours
X67	Intentional self poisoning by and exposure to other gases and vapours
X68	Intentional self poisoning by and exposure to pesticides
X69	Intentional self poisoning by and exposure to other and unspecified chemicals and noxious substances
X70	Intentional self-harm by hanging, strangulation and suffocation
X71	Intentional self-harm by drowning and submersion
X72	Intentional self-harm by handgun discharge
X73	Intentional self-harm by rifle, shotgun and larger firearm discharge
X74	Intentional self-harm by other and unspecified firearm discharge
X75	Intentional self-harm by explosive material
X76	Intentional self-harm by fire and flames
X77	Intentional self-harm by steam, hot vapours and hot objects
X78	Intentional self-harm by sharp objects
X79	Intentional self-harm by blunt objects
X80	Intentional self-harm by jumping from a high place
X81	Intentional self-harm by jumping or lying before moving object
X82	Intentional self-harm by crashing of motor vehicle
X83	Intentional self-harm by other specified means
X84	Intentional self-harm by unspecified means

Source
International Classification of Diseases (ICD-10)

Practitioner classifications

Researchers and clinicians have also attempted to make sense of the self-harm nomenclature by attempting to classify it further. Favazza, an American psychiatrist who has published widely about self-harm, proposed that the behaviour falls into two categories, compulsive and impulsive (Favazza 1996).

Compulsive

Favazza suggested that compulsive self-harm comprises such activities as hair pulling, skin picking and cutting when it is done to remove perceived faults or blemishes in the skin. This behaviour may be ritualistic and carried out by a young person with obsessive compulsive disorder (OCD). For example, the self-harm may be linked to obsessional thoughts and the act relieves tension and relief from thoughts that something bad may happen.

Impulsive

Favazza also refers to impulsive acts of self-harm. Both episodic and repetitive self-harm are impulsive acts, and the difference between them seems to be a matter of degree. Episodic self-harm is self-injurious behaviour engaged in every so often by people who don't think about it otherwise and do not see themselves as self-harmers. What begins as episodic self-harm can escalate into repetitive self-harm, which many practitioners believe should be classified as a separate condition (Kahan and Pattison 1984; Favazza and Rosenthal 1993; Miller 1994).

Self-classification

Practitioners rely heavily on self-reporting by young people. However, some young people are better able to recognise and label their needs and problems than others. The younger the child is, the less developed their insight and self-awareness is likely to be. There are many cognitive and physical changes that take place during adolescence, and the teenage years are characterised by marked mood swings. Young people can be confused about why they self-harm and often struggle to describe their experience. The words and phrases used must always be explored to help ensure that a common understanding and language about the experience of self-harm is reached.

> I suppose I could have told them how rubbish I felt, but I just didn't seem to have the words to describe the absolute despair and pain I was going through.
>
> Kirsty, 17

Myths and legends about self-harm

There are many popular misconceptions about what constitutes self-harm and why young people self-harm. Examining these views and opinions against factual evidence and professional experience can help to frame and come to a better understanding of self-harm and its motivating features. Fox and Hawton have described some of the myths in their book on self-harm in adolescence (Fox and Hawton 2004).

The remaining part of this chapter describes some of the common misconceptions about self-harm. Many of these are not based on any evidence at all, others contradict facts and current professional opinion about the nature of self-harm. Some of what young people think of the myths surrounding self-harm is also discussed. In order to provide the best quality care and optimise recovery, the unhelpful myths and legends about self-harm need to be dispelled and replaced with more balanced social perceptions about self-harm.

'Self-harm is an attempted suicide'

It is rare for self-harm to be an actual suicide attempt. Rather, it can be a way of managing suicidal feelings and it is more often a survival and coping mechanism where the expressed wish may not be to be dead. Self-harming can be a way of regulating strong emotions and brings about tension relief. In some instances, self-harm can be a precursor to suicide. However, this is a much less common phenomenon.

'Self-harm is a teenage girl thing'

The ways in which boys and girls cope with emotions varies, and many boys and young men find it difficult to talk about their feelings. Many prefer to try and cope alone or in silence and refuse to ask for help. It is likely that many more boys self-harm than we know about. Access to help for boys and young men is less well established than support for girls and young women, but some innovative services exist (LifeSigns 2002).

'Females are more likely to kill themselves'

It is true that more girls and young women report that they have considered suicide than boys or young men. However, far more men than women die by suicide each year (Samaritans 2008).

'Young people who self-harm have borderline personality disorder'

People with borderline personality disorder have difficulty controlling their mood, problems in interpersonal relationships, an unstable sense of self and struggle with recognising, understanding, tolerating and communicating emotions. This combination of factors can lead to coping mechanisms, such as self-harm (National Collaborating Centre for Mental Health 2009).

Diagnosing people with borderline personality disorder has historically been a controversial issue. It has been reported that in some cases, being a woman who self-harms is enough to attract such a diagnosis (Spandler and Warner 2007). Needless to say, many people do not find this attitude helpful and seek out services where they feel less judged and more understood.

There is a commonly held myth, particularly amongst professional groups, that borderline personality disorder and self-harm coexist. Believing this misconception to be true can often produce negative outcomes for the young people and their families. Not all people with borderline personality disorder engage in self-harm, and most people who self-harm do not have borderline personality disorder. However, borderline personality disorder is common among adults with chronic self-harming behaviour (Linehan *et al.* 1991; Linehan *et al.* 1999).

Although borderline personality disorder is thought to affect between 0.9 and 3 per cent of young people aged 18 living in the community (Bernstein *et al.* 1993; Lewinsohn *et al.* 1997), the issue of diagnosing young people with this condition is even more contentious than making the diagnosis for adults. NICE has produced guidance on borderline personality disorder which includes children and young people (National Collaborating Centre for Mental Health 2009). The guidance urges practitioners to exercise caution when making a personality disorder diagnosis in young people. This is due to the unstable and developing nature of personality in this age range. However, the guidelines state that borderline personality disorder can be diagnosed for some children under 16. Treatments for self-harm and borderline personality disorder are discussed further in Chapter 7.

'Young people who self-harm are attention seeking ...'

Self-harm is commonly described using negative terms or phrases such as 'attention seeking' or 'manipulative' (Spandler 2001). Generally, it is known that young people who self-harm try to conceal what they are doing rather than draw attention to it. This is because they may feel ashamed, afraid or worried about how other people will react (Barnardo's and Mind 2007).

A national survey of children and young people confirmed that the parents of only 78 of the 248 young people aged 11–15 who said they had hurt themselves were aware of their child's self-harming behaviour (Meltzer *et al.* 2001). One young person told the National Inquiry into self-harm about their perceptions of attention-seeking behaviour:

> Some people do it for attention, like I did when I first started. That doesn't mean they should be ignored. There are plenty of ways to get attention, why cause yourself pain and if someone's crying for help, bloody well give them it, don't stand there and judge the way in which they're asking for it.

The National Inquiry into self-harm also challenges this notion of attention seeking, pointing out that self-harm often takes place in private and
at times is not visible to others (Mental Health Foundation and Camelot
Foundation 2006). In any event, not only is it part of normal human behaviour to seek attention from others, but responsible professionals *should* pay
close attention to a child or young person who is distressed enough to want
to die or hurt themselves.

'... Or manipulative'

In a study of patient views, Nehls (1999) found the view of self-harm as
manipulation to be unfair and illogical, revealing an underlying prejudice and
leading to a negative response to such behaviour by clinicians. Service users in
this study felt it was much more productive and accurate to view self-harm as
a way of controlling emotional pain and not as a deliberate attempt to control
others (Nehls 1999).

Believing self-harm simply to be a matter of manipulation or attention
seeking is unhelpful and misguided, and judgement of this nature should be
avoided. Children and adolescents can find it difficult to explain their self-
harming behaviour, and the response the young person elicits from others is
a crucial factor in therapeutic engagement. Whatever it is, self-harm is an
important communication that the young person has been unable to verbalise
in a less destructive way.

Certainly, at times, the young person may be communicating some unmet
need and may want to elicit help and support, but self-harm is often a private
and hidden concern. It has different meanings for the individual, and encouraging an open discourse about the possible motives is much more helpful than
dismissing the act as manipulative or attention seeking.

Interpreting self-harm accurately is extremely complex and can positively
or negatively affect engagement with the young person. All too often, professionals dismiss the act and view the motives. Their views are frequently
at odds with those of the young person concerned. In the NICE guidelines
on self-harm, young people commented on their negative experiences of
casualty or paediatric wards following self-harm. Young people often felt
that staff did not take their self-harm seriously and dismissed their desire to
die (NICE 2004a).

This is of concern when research has shown that about half of those who
commit suicide had discussed or threatened to kill themselves within 24 hours
of their deaths (Fonagy *et al.* 2002). For this reason, expressions of suicide by
young people should always be taken seriously. The following two quotes
were taken from the National Inquiry report (Mental Health Foundation and
Camelot Foundation 2006) by young people on the issue of attention:

> I had to see a children's psychiatrist, who every week I saw him would tell me I had cut myself for the attention, and asked me why I had wanted the attention. And every week I would tell him why I had really done it and he would never listen. This lack of understanding was so frustrating and patronising, it was supposed to help me stop wanting to cut.

> I was made to sit in a cold corridor while I was waiting for the blood results. The staff were talking about me in the office before that and I could overhear them. 'Time waster – as if we haven't enough to do.' Those words echoed in my head all the next day. I wish they would look closer then they would see me.
>
> Monique, aged 14

A disregard for the young person's distress can reinforce their sense of isolation and failure. Misinterpreting their expression of self-harm or suicide may result in the young person either rejecting offers of help or, worse still, increasing their intent. The young person may have high expectations from professionals involved in their care, hoping that they can provide an instant solution.

Instilling hope for young people who have long since given up is essential, but professionals need to be realistic about what can be offered. The National Inquiry report also reminds us that a non-judgemental and non-blaming approach from practitioners is highly valued by young people.

'Self-harm and suicide is just copycat behaviour'

The Sorrows of Young Werther, written by Goethe in 1774, triggered an increase in suicide leading to its ban in many European states. This became known as the 'Werther Effect' and was to become connected to the origins of the term 'copycat' (Phillips 1974). Today, use of the term copycat is commonly associated with suicides and homicides, or crimes and misdemeanours inspired or replicated by another. Imitation is the process by which one self-harm or suicide attempt exerts a modelling effect on another. Clusters refer to numbers of cases of self-harm or suicides occurring in close proximity with or without any direct link (Blumenthal and Kupfer 1990).

The phenomenon of 'social contagion' is the idea that emotions and behaviours are copied from those around us and can spread rapidly among people and communities. There are many examples of this in everyday life. Yawning, laughing and even the alignment of menstrual cycles of females residing in the same house can be considered as social contagion.

More famous examples of the link between social contagion and suicide come from the history of suicide locations and landmarks. These include Niagara Falls in Canada and Beachy Head on the south coast of England. The Golden Gate Bridge in San Francisco, perhaps the most notorious suicide location in the world, has seen more than 1,300 people jump to their death since it was constructed in the 1930s.

There are many theories about how social contagion works, but as yet no one really understands why (Jones and Jones 1995). The theory can also apply to self-harm and suicide (Rosen and Walsh 1989; Yates 2004). Additional explanatory factors include a combination of grief, over-identification and a fixation on death. This leads to an increase in suicidal behaviour among young people who have been exposed to a suicide (Samaritans 2008).

The media plays an important part in social contagion as it is a means of transmitting or moderating the information which may lead to contagion. At least 60 research studies have explored the relationship between media reporting of suicide and actual suicide, and found that it can lead to imitative behaviours (Blood *et al.* 2007).

There is evidence that the reporting and portrayal of suicide in the media can lead to copycat suicides, especially among young people and those already vulnerable and at increased risk. As the media is so influential on young people and on attitudes in general, there is huge opportunity to educate the public, dispel myths about self-harm and replace these with more accurate information about self-harm and suicide. The National Advisory Council for CAMHS has called on the press to consider their responsibilities when reporting on cases of self-harm and suicide by children and young people (Department for Children, Schools and Families 2008a).

Research has also confirmed that there are issues of social contagion and imitation surrounding young people who self-harm, particularly those who are admitted to inpatient settings (Fox and Hawton 2004). A study by Hawton and colleagues explored the circumstances surrounding self-harm by poisoning by people presenting to accident and emergency services. A fifth of those interviewed reported that a recent television drama in which a leading character took an overdose of paracetamol influenced their own self-harming behaviour (Hawton *et al.* 1999).

As well as concerns about the influence of television, there is growing concern about young people establishing virtual friendships on social networking sites and the use of pro-suicide websites. The role of the mass media in shaping attitudes to self-harm is discussed in Chapter 2. The reality is that a lot of young people communicate with fellow self-harmers using instant messaging, and through international websites such as Bebo, Twitter and Facebook. However, labelling all self-harm as copycat behaviour is very worrying and, in some instances, dangerous. All expressions of self-harm and suicide should be taken seriously and a thorough assessment of risks and needs should be carried out by experienced professionals.

'Self-harming is just a fad'

It is well known that people often do and believe things because many other people do and believe the same things. This is sometimes referred to as the 'bandwagon effect', a phenomenon well documented in the field of behavioural psychology. Since self-harming behaviour is more common among adolescents than any other age group, this leads many to conclude that it is a fad or a phase they are going through.

This may, in part, be true since many young people stop self-harming as they get older and enter adult life. However, for many young people this is not the case, and a small percentage that self-harmed during their adolescent years continue to do so as adults. Some go on to complete suicide. Sound knowledge of risk and protective factors can help professionals more accurately define the risk of those who will go on to complete suicide or suffer adverse psychosocial consequences.

'Young people who talk about suicide never attempt or complete suicide'

Talking about suicidal thoughts can be a plea for help and should always be taken seriously by professionals. Some people believe that talking about suicide, or asking someone if they feel suicidal, will encourage suicide attempts. There is no evidence for this, and failing to ask a suicidal young person how they are feeling may leave them feeling more isolated and unable to express their feelings.

This misconception also reinforces the feelings of shame that young people may be struggling with. Simply ignoring someone's distress can prevent them from getting help at an early stage and may actually increase the chances of a young person harming themselves again. In contrast, talking about suicidal thoughts provides an opportunity for communication and discussion about feelings. Permission to talk about the event can help reduce the feelings of isolation and entrapment.

Many professionals feel anxious about entering into a dialogue with the young person about self-harm or suicide, fearing that it may result in them going on to complete suicide. Again, there is no evidence for this. A number of warning signs may help identify young people who are most at risk. Social withdrawal, lack of concentration and weight loss are each signs that the young person may be depressed. Other young people may externalise their distress and the nature and degree of self-harming behaviours may help inform assessments of a young person's suicidal potential. Risk assessment is discussed later in the book.

'Self-harming through cutting or burning does not hurt those who do it'

Some go a step further and suggest that treatment for self-harm, such as suturing, does not hurt the young person either. They even consider that if a young person is treated in an uncaring manner, this will prevent them self-harming in the future. Consistent reports from service users show that this is nonsense. Although people have different pain thresholds, those who self-harm experience the same sensation of pain as people in general. There is some evidence that when the body experiences injury a group of neurochemicals may lead to a feeling of calm and well-being (Smith *et al.* 1998), but this not the same as saying self-harm does not hurt.

Young people are clear that self-harm from cutting or burning does hurt, and so too can treatment. Potentially painful interventions, such as suturing without appropriate anaesthetic, are unacceptable in modern health care provision and the caring and helping professions. Moreover, practice of this nature is likely to make the young person feel worse, add to their distress and is more likely to increase the chances of them self-harming again. However, because of their negative experience, they may be even less willing to access the health services they need.

The NICE guidelines on self-harm state that young people who have self-injured should be offered adequate anaesthesia and/or analgesia throughout the process of suturing or other painful treatments (NICE 2004a).

'The seriousness of the self-harm can be measured by the severity of the act'

This again is untrue. The seriousness of self-harm cannot be judged purely on the basis of the extent of an injury or size of an overdose. Similarly, the severity of self-harm often has no clear bearing on the degree of distress a young person may be experiencing. Small scratches or cuts or minor acts of self-harm often turn out to be markers of high levels of stress and difficulty.

Some people inaccurately consider that cutting implies low suicidal intent, whereas overdosing is a suicidal act. In fact, both can have lethal consequences and the motives behind both acts can be similar. Certainly, the motives of each young person need to be explored as fully as possible to determine the meaning of the self-harming or suicidal act.

'Young people who self-harm can't be treated'

Young people sometimes report that the need for the helping professions to make things better, often by attempting to stop the self-harm, has the opposite effect. Professionals sometimes become frustrated when their attempts to extinguish the behaviour fail. This can, on occasions, result in the professional taking out their own frustrations on the young person, dismissing them as untreatable.

'Most suicides occur in winter'

Much is written about seasonal affective disorder (SAD), also known as 'winter depression' or 'winter blues'. There is a widespread misconception that suicide rates peak in autumn and winter. This is not true. Instead, most studies confirm that there are more suicides of young people in spring and the summer (Nayha 1982; Partonen *et al.* 2004; Kaledienne *et al.* 2006; Samaritans 2008). Spring and summer peaks have been established in the Northern hemisphere. This has led some to speculate that suicide may be linked to longer and lighter, rather than shorter and darker, days.

Discourse analysis

In moments of desperation, young people who self-harm often express a wish to be dead or take an overdose. This is often shorthand for saying that they are seriously struggling. Parents, friends and professionals naturally want to understand whether the young person is indeed suicidal. The young person may be ambivalent, experiencing conflicting emotions which may intensify at crisis and subside after a difficult experience. Ambivalence is normal. The young person might hate their self-harm, and at the same time recognise that they need it. It is a great help to the young person if the professional is able to understand and accept these changing and conflicting feelings.

Sometimes it is the release of tension that is helpful to young people, as opposed to a desire to bring about death. Undoubtedly, it is a signal of inability to cope with things in that moment. Perhaps not surprisingly, adolescents who are suicidal, and many of those who self-harm, are often more preoccupied by death than other young people. They may write prose and poetry about death and dying, and can lose sight of the irrevocability of death when they are in a psychological crisis. One young person depicted this in a poem entitled 'The End'.

The End, by Katie

I stare into the hole
Wishing back my life that it stole
I slip I fell
Reach out my arm grasps the wall
Blind panic
But I stop, think, consolidate for now
I couldn't live this life anyway
Well I don't see how
Help!
Reality check – my arms now hurt
I stare at my fingers
Clenching the dirt
I begin to release them one by one
Calm throughout
I feel myself drop

I see my life as I go down
As they all say you do
But I smile instead of frown
Watching the memories of happiness that love held
Looking back I feel quite bad
As my body goes
I spot a rope
Like a final plea
Or pearl of hope
I ignore it
Close my eyes
I hear my familiar screams and cries
Guilt takes over me
As I cover my ears
I wish they understood my childish feelings
It's too late now anyway
What is done is done
Drops of tears
Represented by rain
A sign to show the end of pain
Thud
I hit the bottom
Is this it? I wonder
Then the sky darkens
And I see the moon come out
This is the end no doubt
The walls close in
I tingle from within
Smile
Close my eyes
And out loud I say
My final goodbyes
Sorry!

In her poem, Katie describes both an attraction and fear of death. At times throughout her poem death seems the ideal solution, whereas at others she describes panic and guilt. The way that Katie feels about death may depict how she currently feels about her life and discussing the words she has used may assist the professional to engage her and reach a common understanding of what self-harm means. Fantasising about death through her poetry may have been Katie's way of dealing with overwhelming feelings. Instead of wanting to end her life, it may be a way of helping Katie gain a sense of control over her life. For those reading it, however, Katie's poem poses a question about her intentions. It is therefore necessary to inquire about suicidality and intent as part of the engagement process.

Fantasising about suicide is quite common in young people who self-harm. Indeed, it serves as a protective factor from completing suicide. However, fantasy may become less effective as the young person continues to experience feelings of hopelessness and struggles to resolve interpersonal difficulties. Hopelessness, problem solving abilities and skills to resolve conflict need to be considered in order to reach a formulation about intent about self-harm and suicide.

Explaining self-harm

Young people who self-harm often experience difficulty in rationalising and articulating their feelings and behaviours to others. They may not have the emotional vocabulary to describe their thoughts, feelings and intentions. Without these communication skills, distressing issues are likely to be expressed in other ways. If their communication is met with negativity, they may feel further isolated.

Below is an excerpt from a conversation between a professional and a young person that typically denotes the difficulties in understanding self-harm. Tina is aged 14 and has a short-term history of cutting her arms in the context of family difficulties. Emma is a mental-health worker and is talking with Tina on the paediatric ward after deeply cutting her forearm with a razor.

Tina   Not sure why I did it. It seemed the only answer at the time.

Emma   What had been happening, Tina?

Tina   It was just the final straw and I couldn't go on any longer. My thoughts were racing and I wanted to die.

Emma   How long had you been feeling like this?

Tina   I feel like that a lot of the time, like I want to be dead and life is so crap and I know that it's not going to get better. I genuinely wanted to die and get away from things. I have been trying to commit suicide for the last few months.

Emma   Could you tell me a bit about those feelings?

Tina   I just want something to change and I know that by slashing my wrists I will feel calm and when the blood comes out it's just like all the pain is coming out.

Emma   So was it a way of getting rid of all the tension that has been building up?

Tina   I don't know whether I was trying to kill myself or just hurt myself. It's probably impossible to kill yourself that way. Maybe I really just wanted to hurt myself.

From the dialogue you can get a sense of Tina's confusion regarding her self-harm. Intentions are crucial to the psychological meaning of the act. The professional is required to understand the precipitating factors in order to make some sense of what has happened. It is clear that Tina is not sure what she wanted to achieve by cutting herself. Perhaps she was afraid or desperate, which does not encourage clear thinking. Defining the behaviour is often further complicated by ambivalence and uncertainty. Tina appears to be struggling to fathom her own behaviour. She associated her cutting with invoking death, and felt that she had been trying to commit suicide for several months. However, she was able to describe a wish for things to change and sought a release from pain by cutting. She went on to state that it was unlikely that she would die from cutting her wrists and decided that she probably didn't want to die after all.

Summary

There is a lack of clarity and agreement about what defines self-harm and suicidal behaviour, both among those affected by it and those who are involved in helping people with it. Research literature is often no clearer and data analysis makes little difference between fatal self-harm and suicide attempts. It is important to recognise that definitions are far from straightforward. Categories of self-harm and suicide often overlap, descriptors may be used interchangeably, and the intent of young people is frequently changeable or unclear.

The term self-harm is used to describe a young person's behaviour rather than their intent. Therefore, professionals should seek to differentiate self-harming from suicidal behaviour, and terms should remain distinct. More often than not self-harm is not about ending life but is more about regulating emotions, surviving and coping. Although self-harm appears on a spectrum with suicide, each has a different pattern and purpose, and interventions to help have a different foundation and emphasis.

Understanding self-harm requires careful deliberation and the ability to listen respectfully and non-judgementally to exactly what the young person is trying to communicate. Defining their suicidal or self-harming behaviour accurately requires a thorough assessment and a sound understanding of the context in which it is taking place. Reaching a consensus about definitions requires exploration of many factors. These are discussed in depth in the following chapters.

2 Why is self-harm common among young people?

Key points:

- Most self-harm occurs during adolescence. This is an evolving period of physical, psychological and social development, often characterised by confusion, frustration and questions about personal identity. Adolescence involves a shift from dependence to independence and from family to peer groups. For some young people, the transition is difficult and self-harm may be a sign of struggle.
- Research into self-harm has focused on psychosocial factors including stressful life events, alcohol and drug use, child abuse, domestic violence and mental disorder.
- There are many reasons why young people harm themselves. Some do so in an attempt to kill themselves. More commonly, self-harm is not an attempt to die, but a way of dealing with stressful factors, such as bullying or exam pressure.
- The most common problem cited by young people who self-harm is difficult relationships with family members. Problems leading to self-harm can range from persistent arguments and fights, to issues about separation, divorce, parenting and discipline.
- Most young people who self-harm, particularly those who take an overdose, do so impulsively. There is frequently a lack of thought or planning before the self-harm takes place, and little consideration about the consequences.
- Certain groups of young people appear to be at greater risk of self-harm and suicide. These include children who have been sexually abused, those who are looked after by the state, and young people in prison or other secure settings.
- Health professionals must take responsibility for checking their own beliefs and perceptions about self-harm. They must endeavour not to make unhelpful judgements about young people who self-harm, and instead offer them support, understanding and compassion.

Introduction

Young people can feel stressed and unhappy for numerous reasons and it is these experiences that often lead to increased risks of self-harm. Often, the problems young people experience are transient rather than pervasive. Self-harm may be an acute reaction to a one-off situation. The trigger may be an argument with a friend or family member, the end of a relationship between boyfriend and girlfriend or a disappointing exam result.

Self-harm is often an isolated occurrence against the backdrop of a supportive family, understanding and accepting peer group and well developed emotional health and psychological well-being. Young people who self-harm for the first time may feel regret for their actions, want to move on quickly from such an episode and forget it ever happened. However, for other young people, life and their relationships with self-harm is a more complex and persistent problem.

What is the scale of the problem?

The simple answer to this is that we do not know exactly. There are many reasons for this, including poor systems of recognition and recording, and because young people sometimes tell inconsistent stories. One of the major reasons that the prevalence of self-harm cannot be fully known is because many young people who self-harm do so in secret and choose not to tell professionals or other adults. This is sometimes referred to as 'hidden harm'.

Data on suicide is also incomplete, partly because only a very small number of child deaths are registered as suicides; many more child deaths result in open verdicts, or are 'undetermined' or associated with 'misadventure' (McClure 1994; Madge and Harvey 1999). As various researchers have pointed out, failure to accurately estimate the rate of suicide by young people in official figures affects how resources are allocated (Bennewith *et al.* 2005; Sinclair *et al.* 2006; Gosney and Hawton 2007).

The Samaritans was founded in 1953 following the death of a 15-year-old girl who had taken her own life when she started menstruating. She believed that she had contacted a venereal disease. Since this date, the Samaritans volunteers have supported millions of children and young people, including those who are self-harming or suicidal. In 2001 alone, they took over three million calls from people in distress. They estimated that their volunteers explored suicidal feelings with the caller in more than a quarter of these, and the reasons why children and young people were feeling so hopeless varied widely.

Self-harm

A vast amount of research focusing on children and young people who self-harm has been carried out by Professor Keith Hawton and colleagues at the

Oxford University Centre for Suicide Research. It is clear that self-harm by children and young people has increased dramatically in recent decades. Rates of self-harm among British young people are higher than almost all European countries (Hawton *et al.* 1998a).

People who self-harm do not belong to a particular socio-economic or ethnic group, and there are significant differences in incidence and in methods used between men and women. However, Hawton's Oxford study demonstrated that the largest group were females aged 15–24.

The prevalence of self-harm is low in early childhood but rapidly increases during adolescence (Hawton *et al.* 2003). Data from the Office for National Statistics (ONS) shows that as many as one in ten teenagers self-harm, and rates among boys and young men have almost doubled since the 1980s. However, the problem is not restricted to the teenage years. Studies show that a significant number of children aged between five and ten harm themselves (ONS 2006).

Statistics that are collected suggest that 19,000–20,000 young people aged 10–19 are likely to be referred annually to general hospitals in England and Wales following an overdose attempt. About 2,000 are 10–14 years old and the majority are girls (Hawton and Fagg 1992).

The Child and Adolescent Self-harm in Europe (CASE) study is a large multi-centre study across seven countries, including England and Ireland (Madge *et al.* 2008). Over 30,000 young people aged 15–16 completed anonymous questionnaires to indicate whether they had ever harmed themselves. If they had, they were asked to provide further history about their self-harm behaviour. Seventy per cent of those studied admitted to self-harming at some point in their lives. Young people were also asked about their physical and mental health and general lifestyle.

The CASE study found that rates of self-harm were twice as high among girls as boys, and in several countries at least one in ten girls had previously harmed themselves. Around one in five boys and one in four girls remained 'hidden' in the CASE study; that is, they did not go to hospital following self-harm and reported that they did not tell anyone about it.

Although self-harm has been consistently shown to be more common in girls and women across the age range (Shaffer 1974), many boys and young men also harm themselves. Whereas, more young women take non-fatal overdoses of drugs, more young men use violent methods, such as hanging, which is often associated with greater suicidal intent (National Confidential Inquiry into Suicide and Homicide by People with Mental Illness 2009).

Suicide

There is general agreement amongst researchers that suicidal behaviour rises with age, is more common after puberty and increases over the course of adolescence (Woodroffe *et al.* 1993). After road traffic accidents, suicide is the biggest cause of death for young people aged 15–24 (Samaritans 2008).

Data on child and adolescent suicides and undetermined deaths in England and Wales in 2005 reported 184 deaths of young people aged 10–19. Of these, 170 were aged 15–19 (136 males, 34 females), and 14 were aged 10–14 (11 boys, 3 girls) (ONS 2006). In young people aged over 14, suicide is three times more common in boys and young men (17 per 100,000 population) than in girls and young women (5 per 100,000 population) (Samaritans 2008).

What causes self-harm and suicide?

No single factor has been shown to predict self-harm or suicide. However, a combination of external pressures, strong emotions and life events are contributory factors. For some young people, self-harm may be symptomatic of a serious mental health problem such as clinical depression (Pfeffer *et al.* 1991; Brent *et al.* 1994). For others, it may be the result of experimentation and a part of adolescent identity and self-image (Anderson *et al.* 2004).

Triggers include stressful life events and traumatic or abusive experiences, difficulties in relationships and problems at home or school (Social Care Institute for Excellence 2005). Despite popular fantasy, children and young people rarely leave suicide notes to explain their actions. This also makes establishing motives difficult.

Similarly, there is no one reason why self-harm is common among young people. Rather, a combination of individual, family and social factors have led to a huge increase in self-harming behaviours by young people in recent years. It seems the way we are living our lives is leading to an epidemic of mental health problems, which sees self-harm in young people almost become mainstream. If we attempt to visually illustrate causes of self-harm it would look something like Figure 2.1.

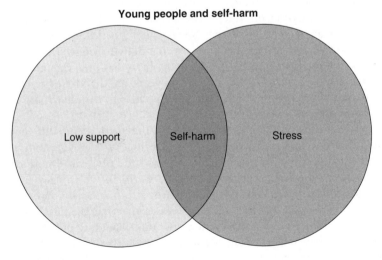

Figure 2.1 Why is self-harm common among young people?

Young people constantly feel under increasing pressure and stress, have inadequate support systems and, by virtue of age, may be less knowledgeable and skilled in adopting healthy coping strategies. Indeed, several studies have shown that a significant proportion of young people who self-harm experience difficulty in solving problems in non-destructive ways and may struggle with difficult and intolerable feelings (McLaughlin *et al.* 1996; Townsend *et al.* 2001). This chapter addresses some of the factors that lead to the scenario proposed in Figure 2.1 and discusses some of the various reasons young people commonly self-harm.

Following an episode of self-harm, clients often report a sense of relief from emotional distress, while others may see it as a way of avoiding dealing with the distress. There are other functions, such as self-punishment and self-regulation. In fact, rather than defining the act, it may be more helpful to ascertain the motivation for the act. Getting the young person to discuss triggers and events surrounding their self-harm will aid definition, and subsequently treatment.

Adolescence

An understanding of adolescent development is an essential normative anchor point when working with young people who self-harm. The nature of adolescence has been debated over many years, and is the transitional stage between childhood and adulthood. The health and welfare of adolescents has received increasing attention in the last decade. This is largely because adolescents make up 13–15 per cent of the UK population (RCPCH 2003), and because adolescence is a period of physical, psychological and social growth. Adolescents are also large consumers of health services. Although it is commonly believed that most young people are healthy, more than half will visit their GP at least once every year, and approximately 30 per cent have some type of chronic health problem (Coleman *et al.* 2007).

Despite the growing interest in the health and welfare of young people, there is little agreement about the age at which a child becomes an adolescent, the factors and developmental tasks that define adolescence or when an adolescent becomes an adult. Historically, puberty has been thought to mark the onset of adolescence. However, in recent years, children have been starting puberty at a younger age which makes the periods of childhood and adolescence more difficult to discern.

As a social construct, adolescence means different things to different people and the concept varies across cultures. During this period, young people experiment, question and try to make sense of the physical, emotional and social changes affecting their lives and the world in which they live. The transitional phase of adolescence takes place within a social context. Being aware of this, as well as wider social processes affecting the development of the individual, may help us achieve a deeper understanding of the issues that impact to produce self-harm (Anderson *et al.* 2004). Erikson (1968) has been influential in understanding adolescent psychological development which includes the attainment of several key tasks:

- independence
- the formation of sexual role and orientation
- self-control of aggressive and oppositional impulses
- achievement of adolescent identity.

While there will always be individual differences according to temperament and personality traits, for some adolescents experimentation can include participating in risky behaviours. This is often with the aim of wanting to have fun and, in the absence of danger or negative consequences, these risky behaviours are often seen as normal in the context of adolescent development (Kloep and Hendry 1999).

Risk taking

In their book on alcohol, drugs, sex and youth, Plant and Plant (1992) suggest that risk taking is a characteristic of normal adolescent development and behaviour. For example, hanging on to the back of a bus or lorry, jumping into water off a ledge, lighting fires or running across railway tracks are not uncommon behaviours among young people.

However, when things go wrong and young people and others are injured or die as a result, these behaviours are rightly condemned as irresponsible and foolhardy. It has been suggested that the majority of these risky behaviours are carried out by boys, and it is reported that few move from experimental to chronic risk taking (Moore and Parsons 2000). However, the most common reason for hospital admission of boys during adolescence is for head injuries and open wounds (Coleman *et al.* 2007).

Another problem facing adolescents is their oppression within multiple social contexts. Young people lack power because of their age, size and lack of access to resources. This is in addition to other factors that may disadvantage them, such as socio-economic class, race and gender. Young people react to such oppression in a number of ways. This includes passive acceptance, using illegitimate coercive power or manipulation of peers and retaliation (Kingston *et al.* 2004). There are a number of proximal and distal explanations for why adolescents may engage in self-harming or suicidal behaviours:

Precipitating factors

- retaliation against real or perceived wrongs
- relief or escape from unbearable pain
- to distract family from another issue
- reunion fantasies, e.g. joining sibling or parent
- an attempt to gain control over their lives
- humiliating experience
- pregnancy
- break-up with peers.

Predisposing factors

- lack of boundaries, structure and direction
- intense pressure to succeed
- publicised suicide
- history of suicide in family or friendship circles
- family discord, poor communication, lack of cohesive values.

It may seem obvious that when working with a young person who has self-harmed, their behaviour needs to be understood in the context of adolescent development, which is a time of rapid physical, psychological and social changes.

Independence

The journey through adolescence and towards adulthood usually involves a change in relationships with parents or carers. Young people have an increasing need for privacy, both physically and emotionally, and embark on a drive to become independent and self-sufficient. Whereas younger children often share worries and concerns with parents and carers, this is less likely to happen during adolescence when there develops a shift towards the peer group as a source of support.

This developmental stage is not always straightforward for some young people. A belief that problems must be resolved without the support of adults may lead some to struggle. Indeed, a large survey showed that parents are often unaware that their child is self-harming at all (Meltzer *et al.* 2001).

Impulse control

As adolescence progresses, young people usually become better able to control their impulses and emotions. This not only takes longer for some than others to achieve, but some young people also find it a difficult developmental task to master. Perhaps not surprisingly, self-harm is more prevalent during adolescence when young people are less skilled and experienced in managing their impulses and strong emotions.

Research confirms this hypothesis. Ample evidence has indicated that self-regulation, such as the ability to control impulses, tends to deteriorate during periods of emotional distress. Most young people who self-harm, particularly those who take an overdose, do so impulsively (Skegg 2005). There is frequently a lack of thought or planning before the self-harm takes place, and little consideration about the consequences.

Half the participants in the CASE study reported that they had harmed themselves within an hour of the episode in question (Madge *et al.* 2008). In addition, a self-report survey in schools found that adolescents who were more impulsive and had a negative self-regard were at greater risk of self-harm. However, impulsivity was not shown to be an independent risk factor for boys

(Hawton *et al.* 2002). Favazza and Rosenthal (1993) argue the case for repetitive self-mutilation (RSM) to be classified as an impulse control disorder.

Sexuality and personal identity

The increased reliance on friends to provide a model on how to behave leads the young person to position themselves in a group of like-minded people. They experience a growing pressure to conform, to look good, to fit in and develop relationships. Adolescence is a time of identity formation, and teenagers are working out who they are and who they want to become.

During adolescence, young people often 'try out' different identities as part of their journey to 'find out who they are'. Puberty also impacts on their body image, with which they can become temporarily more preoccupied. For young people who are in the process of forging a constructive sense of identity, positive experiences of sexual expression and intimate relationships can help validate their sense of self-worth. In comparison, negative experiences may lead to guilt, shame and a sense of worthlessness.

Of course, it is not just friends who are influential. Family play a role in the acceptance or rejection of a young person's sexuality. Society also plays a critical part in defining socially acceptable values and norms, and this can be particularly evident during adolescence. Young people may feel confused about their sexuality, as lots of people have feelings for someone of the same sex at some stage in their life. However, this is a natural part of sexual development and the formation of self-identity.

Some young people struggle with this process more than others and worry that their feelings may be abnormal. Just as adolescence is a period of transition, so too is the development of sexuality and self-identity. While young people should not feel under pressure to label their sexuality, those who are clear about their sexual orientation should be supported to express this without feeing marginalised.

Lesbian, gay and bisexual young people

Young people who are lesbian, gay or bisexual are vulnerable, not because of their sexual orientation, but because of their lack of acceptance and the experiences of discrimination and stigma they often face. Growing up around other young people who are forming their own views, both positive and negative, about sexuality and sexual identity may be a difficult and challenging process.

Research has shown that young people are at increased risk of experiencing discrimination and social exclusion if they are attracted to the same sex (Mental Health Foundation and Camelot Foundation 2006). For young people who are gay and do not feel safe in 'coming out', fear of rejection can lead to self-harm (Brown 2002).

Although there is a lack of robust evidence, young people who are lesbian, gay or bisexual may be more vulnerable to self-harm and suicide. Research has suggested that girls who are worried about their sexual orientation are four times more likely to report self-harm than girls without these concerns. In comparison, boys worried about their sexual orientation are twice as likely as other males to report harming themselves (Hawton and Rodham 2006a). It is therefore important to consider issues of gender and sexual orientation as part of the assessment and helping process.

Stress and resilience

Resilience is the capacity to cope with life's challenges and is both psychological and physical. Some children are able to grow and flourish in the most adverse circumstances and have been called 'dandelion children'. Others are less resilient and more like orchids – they suffer in harsh environments but may thrive in a climate of care and support (Thomas-Boyce and Ellis 2005). This is partly genetic, but resilience is also dependent on a number of personal, environmental, social and experiential factors (Williams 2008).

The capacity for resilience grows and develops over time, and is enhanced and threatened by factors within the individual and wider social system. While there is a greater focus on the peer group during adolescence, the family remains an important source of support in terms of building resilience as the young person moves towards adulthood and independence.

A positive child–parent attachment involving warmth, encouragement, care and understanding is the basis for a secure and supportive relationship. This caring relationship, along with non-judgemental, high expectation messages and opportunities for participation and contribution, promotes emotional health and well-being in the young person.

This resilience, in turn, helps protect against risks, such as engaging in self-harm, as a way of coping with stress. In their excellent book, Daniel and Wassell (2002) provide a summary of the factors associated with resilience in children. These include being:

- female
- sociable
- independent
- reflective rather than impulsive
- able to express emotions.

As well as having:

- hobbies
- a sense of humour
- a willingness and capacity to plan
- good communication skills
- empathy with others
- a sense of competence and being able to do things for oneself

- problem solving skills
- autonomy.

However, not all young people grow up in an emotionally supportive climate. Some are at higher risk of self-harm due to negative experiences during childhood. The psychological resilience they need in order to deal with the developmental tasks of adolescence is either lacking or poorly developed.

This may mean that experience of problems is more intense or pervasive, and the risk of self-harm is increased as a consequence. Research consistently highlights a number of factors which threaten resilience and lead to increased rates of self-harm (Ross and Heath 2002), and these are discussed throughout this book.

Pressure to succeed

Many young people are under intense pressure to succeed. This is from parents, teachers and friends. These pressures may peak around the time of exams or be associated more generally with coursework. Young people may self-harm after getting lower grades than predicted, or may harm themselves more regularly as a way of coping with the demands of school and the level of work expected.

Attention seeking

No discourse on self-harm would be complete without an attempt to grapple with the derogatory term 'attention seeking'. It is part of human nature that children and young people seek and need attention. As social beings we need social interaction, feedback and validation of our worth. This is part of the psychological maturation process and the development of what some refer to as 'emotional intelligence' (Mayer *et al.* 2008).

Very often, young people who self-harm are looking for positive attention they are not getting in their lives. In an attempt to challenge some of the myths and stigma about self-harm, some professionals have replaced the phrase 'attention seeking' with 'attention needing'. This shifts the emphasis from a young person doing something 'wrong' to someone else's responsibility to do something 'right'. Self-harm, of course, does not happen to a person in isolation. It is relational, has a social context and is influenced by the system in which the young person lives.

> The self-harm made me feel important ... it got me noticed and taken seriously at school.
>
> Ellie, 15

Youth subculture

As stated earlier, many behaviours during adolescence are not usually regarded as self-harm. However, with the 'experimental' phase of adolescence in mind, it is easy to see how self-harm might be something which is tried and tested. In discussing the relative emotional coping strategies of boys and girls, Hawton (1986) suggests that girls tend to be more 'intro-punitive' than boys in expressing their distress. By this he means that girls are more likely to self-harm than boys, who are more likely to engage in the high-risk behaviour described earlier.

Many young people will self-harm once and not self-harm again, but others will continue for a variety of different reasons, which are explored later in this chapter. Some young people self-harm as part of a social group. Over the years, there have been examples of youth cultures that include self-harm in their identity. Goth has been described as a subgenre of punk with a dark and sinister aesthetic, with aficionados conspicuous by their range of distinctive clothing and make-up and tastes in music (Hodkinson 2002).

A study of 1,258 young people identified as goths was undertaken in Scotland by Young and colleagues. They found that belonging to the goth subculture was strongly associated with lifetime self-harm and attempted suicide, with a prevalence of 53 per cent and 47 per cent respectively, among the most highly identified group (Young *et al.* 2006). More recently, 'emos', short for emotional, have been associated with self-harm. Indeed, part of emo culture includes the display of visible scars and celebration of self-harm. However, it is important to state that not all young people who call themselves goths or emos self-harm.

Young people are on their way to achieving a number of developmental tasks during adolescence. These include the attainment of independence, self-control of aggressive and oppositional impulses, and the construction of individual sexuality and identity. These present young people with a range of issues and challenges which are discussed in turn.

Family relationships

The most common problem cited by young people who self-harm is difficult relationships with family members. In a large survey of children under 15, over three-quarters stated that problems in the family were their primary concern (Hawton and Harriss 2008). Problems leading to self-harm can range from persistent arguments and fights to issues about separation, divorce, parenting and discipline.

Young people who have self-harmed also report that loss through a family bereavement or breakdown in a relationship is often a source of stress. Not only do they miss the person who has died or left, but other members of the family who are usually supportive may be struggling with their own feelings of loss and sadness and are less available to support the young person.

Some young people say that they feel unloved or that they feel different to others members of the family. This sometimes manifests as emptiness or a sense of not belonging. Whether they have people around them or not, some young people feel lonely. This perceived or real lack of connection with parents or other family members may be a transitional phase, but for some it represents more severe attachment difficulties and young people may feel isolated and at greater risk of self-harm. Anniversaries of losses experienced by young people can also be significant for those who self-harm.

Looked After Children

A particularly vulnerable group of young people are those who are 'looked after' by the local authority and who live with foster carers or in residential children's homes (HM Government 2008). By nature of their looked-after status, their relationship with parents has been considered troubled enough to instigate safeguarding concerns about their welfare. This may be about their parent's ability to actually parent – to look after, care, protect and appropriately control the young person – and where they are not able to do this, sometimes there is a need to protect the young person from their own behaviour that is putting them at risk of significant harm.

Research from Northern Ireland has confirmed that children looked after by the state show higher rates of self-harm and suicidal behaviour (Brodie *et al.* 1997; Cousins *et al.* 2008). A review of the circumstances surrounding 50 looked after children who died during a four-year period concluded that 11 were completed suicides (Scottish Executive 2002b). A small follow-up study of 48 care leavers showed that 17 (35 per cent) had self-harmed and 29 (60 per cent) had thought about, or attempted, suicide (Saunders and Broad 1997).

Ironically, once in residential care, by putting a group of the most vulnerable young people together, other factors, such as social contagion, may come into play, so if a young person has not self-harmed previously, they are at increased risk of doing so (Christofferson *et al.* 2003). This is discussed further later in this chapter. To help meet the mental health needs of young people in care, many CAMHS teams now include Looked After Children (LAC) professionals. These professionals provide regular consultation and support to young people and staff in residential children's homes and foster care. This may include a focus on a young person's self-harming behaviour, or support for the staff or carers in meeting the needs of young people on a day to day basis.

Payne and Butler (2003) drew attention to the fact that looked after children represent one per cent of the total child population, but account for ten per cent of those who present with self-harm to accident and emergency departments. The National Inquiry recommended that there is a need for more research to find out why certain environments such as children's residential or secure settings seem to be more likely to trigger self-harm, and what can be done to change these environments (Mental Health Foundation and Camelot Foundation 2006).

Black and ethnic minority young people

Britain is a multicultural society with one in eight people belonging to an ethnic minority community. Disadvantage, discrimination and inequalities in mental health are of particular concern among ethnic minority groups. Increased rates of self-harm, suicide attempts and completed suicide have been reported in some groups of young people. It is of concern that the rate of suicide for Asian women in England and Wales is three times higher than for women of white British origin (Raleigh and Balarajan 1992; Avan and Bakshi 2004).

There are likely to be several reasons for these trends. Gender discrimination, racism and domestic violence are all contributory factors (Glasgow Violence Against Women Partnership 2008). The concepts of 'izzat', meaning 'honour', and 'sharam', meaning 'shame', derive from Pakistan and the Indian subcontinent. These cultural concepts affect how girls and women dress, behave, and who they can talk to, be friends with or marry. Izzat can be both influential and a source of pressure for some British Asian girls and young women. In a focus group of young women aged 16–25, some felt that to protect izzat it would be better to commit suicide than leave an abusive relationship (Gilbert *et al.* 2004).

Research from the Newham Asian Women's Project (NAWP) found that young Asian women were two to three times more vulnerable to self-harm than their non-Asian counterparts. However, NAWP highlight the need to look beyond the notion that cultural conflict is the main reason for such high rates of self-harm and suicide. Whilst recognising that self-harm allows young Asian women to maintain the notion held by their community and culture that problems should stay within the family and that it is not acceptable to seek outside help, it is important to address the more fundamental factors that lead to self-harm and suicide. These include racism, sexism, class inequality, patriarchy, sexual abuse, violence and immigration.

To address these problems, NAWP has developed the *Zindaagi Mental Health Project* for young Asian women vulnerable to self-harm and suicide. 'Zindaagi', meaning 'life', aims to promote education and awareness about self-harm and break down the taboos and stigma that are associated with the problem. The project involves outreach counselling, a teenagers' group and early intervention in schools. *Zindaagi* also works with faith leaders to raise awareness and to direct young women towards help and support services. However, the uptake of mental health services by black and ethnic minority young people remains low (Neale *et al.* 2005). This may be partly due to prejudiced, stereotyped and racist perceptions that have permeated through mental health service planning and delivery.

Husain *et al.* (2006) has suggested that early intervention in schools and the transitional phase during adolescence may be an ideal opportunity to explore gender role expectations, individual and cultural conflict as a means of preventing the sudden and significant increased risks in the years after leaving school.

Trauma and abuse

Many children and young people who self-harm have backgrounds characterised by emotional, physical and sexual abuse (Green 1978; Romans *et al.* 1995; Santa Mina and Gallop 1998; Gladstone *et al.* 2004; Social Care Institute for Excellence 2005). However, it is important to state that not all those who self-harm have been abused as children, and that not all young people who have suffered abuse self-harm. Further research is needed on the link between abuse and neglect, including emotional neglect, and self-harm (National Collaborating Centre for Women's and Children's Health 2009).

Brown *et al.* (1999) studied a cohort of 776 randomly selected children over a 17-year period from 1975–92 and concluded that children who had a history of sexual abuse were at greater risk of becoming depressed or suicidal during their adolescence and young adulthood. A history of sexual abuse was also found to be one of the risk factors for self-harm in a study conducted by Vajda and Steinbeck (1999), who undertook a retrospective medical record review of adolescents 13 and 20 years old who presented at the emergency department.

Young people who have experienced isolated incidents of abuse, such as rape, may harm themselves because they feel shame, anger or confusion. Self-harm may be an expression of self-disgust or self-punishment (Ainscough and Toon 1998). Whilst responsibility for sexual abuse always lies with the perpetrator, their victims frequently experience a sense of guilt and responsibility and often blame themselves. Young people may also use self-harm to cope with keeping their experiences of abuse secret, or to help cope with any subsequent investigations into abuse. Police statements, physical examination and court appearances are themselves stressful and young people may harm themselves to cope with what is a mentally and physically intrusive process.

As well as historical abuse, a child or young person may be currently being abused. Children who are being sexually abused often experience a sense of powerlessness; their bodies and feelings are invaded and violated and they are unable to protect themselves or control what is happening to them (Ainscough and Toon 1998). Young people frequently attempt to take control back in some way, and this can be enabled through self-harm. An act of self-harm may also become protective or self-preserving. For example, hospitalisation following an overdose may temporarily prevent further abuse from happening because the young person is in a safe place and cannot be accessed by their abuser.

It is important to recognise that abuse is often carried out in families, by caregivers who should be in a position of trust. Sometimes the abuse has occurred in the past and is known by the family. At other times, the young person may have kept their abuse secret. They may have been struggling with intense negative experiences and decide to tell someone during the assessment or when talking to family or friends. A thorough assessment of childhood trauma, self-harm behaviours, suicidal ideation and suicide attempts is necessary to help identify young people at greatest risk, and so that needs can be identified and addressed.

The Basement Project provides support for people who have been abused as children and those who self-harm. The project also provides training, supervision and consultation for workers in community and mental health services and has published a range of useful resources and training materials (Basement Project 1997).

Domestic violence

Asking young people who self-harm about their experiences of past or present abuse is seen as good clinical practice, but it is also important to specifically ask young people about their experiences of domestic violence as they may not otherwise share this information. At least 750,000 children a year witness domestic violence (Department of Health 2002a). How they respond to and cope with this trauma depends on a range of factors including age, sex and stage of development. According to the Royal College of Psychiatrists (RCP) the effects of witnessing domestic violence can include self-harm by taking overdoses or cutting (RCP 2004a).

Young people who have experienced domestic violence often experience mental health difficulties such as anxiety and depression. Many young people experience fear and distress and psychological and behavioural problems that are not always recognised or understood to be associated with domestic violence (Worrall *et al.* 2008). The relationship between self-harm and abuse, and the association between self-harm and domestic violence suggests that early detection and protection could reduce the need for people to self-harm later in life (NICE 2004a).

Bullying

Bullying was the biggest single reason for children and young people calling ChildLine in 2007, representing 18 per cent of their calls (NSPCC 2008a). The impact of bullying on children's mental health, emotional well-being and general development cannot be overstated. It takes many forms and ranges from name calling, to direct physical attacks, and includes spreading rumours, social exclusion and isolation, threats of violence and destruction of the victim's property. Bullying can also include racial or sexual discrimination.

It is not unusual for children and young people who are bullied to become anxious, depressed and refuse to attend school (Woolley 2006). Whilst the effects of bullying are generally agreed to be emotionally harmful, some young people manage to cope and are not unduly affected or distressed. A supportive network of friends and family and sensitive school based interventions are likely to be protective factors. For others however, bullying may be serious, persistent or cause psychological or physical harm. Young people may fear serious injury, feel humiliated and out of control and self-harm in desperation.

> They would all make fun of me. Called me psycho bitch and emotional. The teachers tried to help but most of it happens when they are not around.

Several independent inquiries into the suicide of young people have high-lighted bullying as a significant causative factor. For example, a spate of deaths of young soldiers at Deepcut Barracks in Surrey during the late 1990s resulted in significant media interest and speculation about bullying as well as concern about access to weapons by vulnerable young people (Cathcart 2007).

It is not unusual for bullying to be done by a former close friend, some-one with whom a young person had trusted and shared personal information. Young people tell us that this leaves them feeling betrayed and vulnerable to further bullying.

> However self-harm is tackled within schools or anywhere else, if they didn't make it such a dirty subject, people would come forward a lot more quickly to get help.

When bullying takes place at school, having to attend and face the bullies can be extremely difficult. The government has made tackling bullying in schools a key priority. All state schools are required to have anti-bullying policies and procedures and have been issued with anti-bullying packs based on legisla-tion, recent research and good practice (Department for Education and Skills 2002). School programmes have been initiated which include awareness rais-ing, assertiveness training, peer support and mentoring. Despite this, young people often feel unsupported by teachers and many complain bitterly about the inept strategies that have been adopted by schools.

> Just because I am not an 'It Girl' they think I'm a freak. One girl started making gestures like she was cutting her arm and another put a razor in my PE kit. The teachers were aware of what was going on but they didn't know how to tackle the girls. I used to wish it would stop and that the new teacher would be the one who would rescue me.

In some cases, young people feel their only option is to change schools. Sometimes young people self-harm as a means of communicating the extent of their distress to those around them. They want parents and teachers to know that they are struggling to cope with the situation. Parents often report that they are aware that their son or daughter has self-harmed, but go on to say that they had no idea that the problems were so serious. It seems tragic that young people have to go to such extremes to get people to listen and help them.

In recent years, the proliferation of social networking and virtual friendships has led to the growth of 'cyber bullying'. This has been linked to self-harm and suicide by young people, including the well-publicised suicide of Megan Meier, a 13-year-old girl from the USA. Megan hanged herself after being bullied on MySpace. The case caused several of the US jurisdictions to enact or consider legislation prohibiting harassment over the Internet. In the UK, *Respect Me*, Scotland's anti-bullying service, has attempted to respond to the problem by issuing guidance on cyber bullying. This includes information on how to encourage the responsible use of technologies, important points to discuss with children and young people and additional points for parents, carers and organisations.

Young people in secure settings

The mental health needs of children and young people in local authority secure children's homes (LASCH) and prisons are known to be considerable, severe and complex, with rates of psychosis, self-harm and suicide well above those of other children (Utting 1997; Department of Health 2007a). The prevalence of self-harm by adult women in prison is high, but for young people in prison the rates are twice as high (Youth Justice Board 2006).

This is partly explained by the high prevalence of psychosocial adversity experienced by young people in secure settings, including substance misuse, child abuse and mental disorder, which are themselves risk factors for self-harm (Singleton *et al.* 1998). In a study of girls in custody who had offended, Wilkinson *et al.* (2002) found that most girls were extremely vulnerable, poor, had been sexually or physically abused and had self-harmed.

However, rates of self-harm are also high as a result of being in a secure setting. The shock and physical and emotional isolation of custody leaves young people additionally vulnerable. Young people frequently report feeling unsafe and may experience bullying and exploitation in custody (Utting 1997; Bradley 2009). In a sample of 73 young women held in secure settings, over one-third had self-harmed in the previous month. The majority (93 per cent) told researchers they had cut themselves to relieve feelings of anger, tension, anxiety and depression, rather than draw attention to their situation. For the minority who had harmed themselves, several had witnessed other young people cutting.

Arrival in custody is often the time when young people are at greatest risk of self-harm or suicide (HM Inspectorate of Prisons 2007). In a joint report for the Ministry of Justice and Department for Children, Schools and Families, young people in secure settings have also reported that responses to their self-harm are often punitive, including segregation and physical restraint (Smallridge and Williamson 2008). The following excerpt is taken from a report by the Youth Justice Board (2006) and illustrates the difficulties facing young people in secure settings:

> Basically, when my Nan died I started on the road, drinking and smoking crack. I went a bit loopy and stuff. I started self-harming, just doing little scratches and that. Then when I got sent to jail, I found out my boyfriend had been involved in a car crash and he was on a life support machine. I had to go and turn it off and that sent me a bit more over the edge. I just decided to do big cuts on my arms and on my stomach and that. I've tried killing myself about seven times, overdosed and stuff just because I feel my life's not worth living at the moment. My little girl's been taken into care and I just feel like self-harming most of the time.

It is not only rates of self-harm that are high among young people in secure settings. In addition, suicide by children and young people in custody is a major concern and there have been numerous deaths of young people by suicide in the UK in the last decade.

Alcohol and drugs

The number of young people consuming excessive amounts of alcohol has grown enormously in recent years (Rossow *et al.* 2007). MacLachlan and Smyth (2004) report growing concern towards a binge drinking and youth culture where young people regularly consume large quantities of alcohol. There is evidence that the alcohol and drug scenes are merging because both are now freely available to young people (Institute of Alcohol Studies 2006).

Young people report that alcohol and drug use makes them feel relaxed, explore sexual relationships and increase confidence. The reasons young people give for drinking alcohol are similar to those reported surrounding self-harm. These include coping with stress, wanting to feel better, and altering a mood state. Alcohol and drug misuse was reported in 14 per cent of young people presenting to hospital for the first time following self-harm (Hawton *et al.* 2003). This figure is likely to have increased more recently as the use of alcohol by young people grows.

Mental health problems

Self-harm is not classified as a mental disorder, and most agree that it is often a symptom and manifestation of significant unmet needs. It can exist with other problems or be a symptom of other disorders. Some young people who self-harm may have more serious underlying mental health problems, such as depression, psychosis or eating disorders (Webb 2002).

In particular, self-harm has been associated with emotional and behavioural disorders among children and young people. ONS data on 7,404 children aged 5–15 found that 324 had an emotional disorder and 355 had a conduct disorder (Green *et al.* 2005). The international CASE study examined depression and anxiety and found that the risk of emotional disorders was highest in those who had either thought of harming themselves, or had done so, than among those who had not (Madge *et al.* 2008).

> It keeps me happy in front of others. It stops my depression spilling out.

Self-harming and suicidal behaviour can also be associated with eating disorders, such as anorexia nervosa, bulimia disorder and binge eating disorder (Favazza *et al.* 1989; Thomas *et al.* 2002; Sansone and Levitt 2002). A number of common characteristics of young people struggling with both eating disorders and self-harm have been identified. These include dissociation and impulsivity.

Hopelessness

Hopelessness and despair have been described as the missing link between depression and suicide. In addition, a sense of hopelessness in young people is a known risk factor for self-harm (Hawton and James 2005). McLaughlin *et al.* (1996) suggest that hopelessness as part of adolescent self-harm is an important independent variable over and above depression. In their study, young people reported a wide range of problems associated with family relationships, school and problem solving (McLaughlin *et al.* 1996).

It is therefore important that health professionals talk with young people about their hopes and ideas for the future and explore any hopelessness. Encouraging young people to have goals and aspirations and supporting them to achieve these fosters hope and purpose. Whilst important for all young people, this is crucial for those who may struggle to achieve in a society where there is increasing pressure to perform academically or vocationally. Hopelessness is not just associated with education and unemployment, but is influenced and developed through supportive relationships, hobbies and interests, and a sense of purpose in life.

Inadequate support

As part of a self-harm assessment we often ask young people where their ideas to self-harm came from. However, if self-harm has been impulsive the young person may not have a clear idea of how they got into the situation. Yet, when asked if they know anyone who has self-harmed, very often young people do. They may be aware of someone in their immediate or extended family, a close friend or just know about a person at school or in the community, illustrating that self-harm is very common.

Stigma

Despite publicity raising the profile of mental health and campaigns focused on reducing stigma, people are often reluctant to speak about their own struggles with self-harm, believing this may adversely affect their profile or career opportunities. Indeed, in going public and telling people about their experiences, they may be unfairly judged or discriminated against. Therefore, self-harm often remains a secret as people feel ashamed, guilty and think that they should not talk about it.

This has huge implications for young people who want and need help, but feel unable to access it. Although self-harm has now become so common it is almost mainstream, many young people feel alone, reluctant and unwilling to confide in others (Mental Health Foundation and Camelot Foundation 2006).

Of course, some people choose not to share their experiences of self-harm (Ystgaard *et al.* 2009). Many will remember the 1995 BBC television interview with the late Princess Diana who shocked the world by admitting she cut her arms and legs and had thrown herself down a flight of stairs on more than one occasion. Famously, the princess said:

> You have so much pain inside yourself that you try and hurt yourself on the outside because you want help.

In another interview, Diana revealed that she started self-harming due to the pressure she felt trying to adapt to her role as Princess of Wales, but said that it backfired as rather than getting the help she needed, it made people think she was attention seeking and unstable. It has been suggested that help-seeking by people who self-harm increased following Princess Diana's disclosure (Austin and Kortum 1996). So, too, however, did rates of suicide in the months that followed Diana's death (Hawton *et al.* 2000).

The NICE guidelines on self-harm state that as a matter of good practice, people who self-harm should be treated with the same care, respect and privacy as any patient (NICE 2004a). That this even needs to be stated is evidence that discrimination and stigma are experienced by people who self-harm and who are not already routinely treated in this way. Public health strategies to reduce stigma are discussed further in Chapter 10.

Suicide, crime and faith

The historical legal position on suicide has not helped public perceptions, having historically been treated as a criminal matter in many parts of the world. It was considered a criminal offence in England until the Suicide Act was passed in 1961, and until as recently as 1993 in the Republic of Ireland. Regarding suicide as an offence can sometimes bring shame and embarrassment and people who have killed themselves are treated accordingly. Whilst the family and friends of a person who had died by suicide were trying to understand how this situation had come about, rather than a culture of compassion and understanding was an environment of blame and humiliation. Many people therefore discourage the phrase 'committing suicide' since the term 'commit' is most frequently associated with crime.

Historically, there have also been additional consequences of suicide depending on religious beliefs. In most forms of Christianity, suicide is considered a sin, although it is sometimes believed that mental illness or grave fear of suffering diminishes the responsibility of the person completing suicide. In ancient Greece, a person who had committed suicide (without the approval of the state) was denied the honours of a normal burial. They would be buried in a simple grave, away from the city and without a headstone or other marker. Christian burials and funerals of people who had died by suicide were also denied. Instead they had to be buried in unconsecrated ground. A criminal ordinance issued by Louis XIV in 1670 confirmed the attitudes of the day to suicide. The dead person's body was drawn through the streets, face down, and then hung or discarded on a rubbish heap. All their previous property was confiscated by the state. In India, attempted suicide is a crime punishable by imprisonment.

Suicide attacks were carried out by Japanese kamikaze air pilots during the Second World War, and, today, suicide bombers commit acts of terrorism in some parts of the world. At the time of writing this book, children in Palestine, Iraq and Afghanistan are killing themselves by detonating bombs strapped to suicide vests. Notwithstanding the overarching safeguarding concerns, these issues illustrate the complex interrelationship between faith and suicide and the different reasons why young people kill themselves.

Even today, UK insurance companies often have suicide clauses built into their policies. For example, some state that claims can only be made if the policy was open for more than two years prior to the death by suicide. Given the legal backdrop and the perceived relationship between self-harm and suicide it is perhaps not surprising that stigma persists. It is important to be aware that cultural issues may influence a young person's willingness to seek help.

Coping strategies

Each of us has differing abilities at different times to use safe and healthy coping strategies. We all face stress and adversity at some point in our lives, but for some these pressures are much greater than for others. As Williams (2008) points out, too many children and young people grow up with challenges and seriously adverse circumstances with which they cannot deal alone. When this happens to young people who have not yet developed stress management and conflict resolution skills, they may encounter problem solving difficulties and not know where to turn. Adolescence brings with it additional challenges, and problems may feel magnified by young people whose bodies and minds are undergoing many simultaneous changes.

Babiker and Arnold (1997) suggest that people who self-harm have often found a behaviour that provides a singularly powerful solution to the problem of expressing or coping with overwhelming feelings. Supporting a young person to expand their interpersonal and cognitive skills gradually enables them to consider and evaluate different strategies. McLaughlin *et al.* (1996) found that many young people who self-harm were unable to generate solutions to their problems; they could not find different ways out of the difficulties which lead to their self-harm. Often, the task of therapy is to assist them to replace self-harm with non-destructive coping strategies. A clear and consistent message from young people is that simply trying to get them to stop self-harming is usually ineffective in itself (Mental Health Foundation and Camelot Foundation 2006).

> Don't tell them to stop – they could get worse because it's their way of coping. You need to put the structure in first. Otherwise it's like leaving a baby alone without food and water.

Equally unhelpful, is entering into agreements where young people are asked to promise not to self-harm. This can put a lot of emotional pressure on them and may add to feelings of guilt and betrayal they may already be struggling with. For some young people, self-harm is their only coping strategy. If it is removed, they have nothing.

Young people and social identity

Politicians, sociologists and the lay public are concerned that the culture of immediate access to material goods and friends has seen a decreasing sense of community in the UK. Families have become more mobile, more mothers are working and community facilities are closing. People tend to keep to themselves rather than foster a shared sense of responsibility. Instead of talking to young people in the neighbourhood and getting to know them, adults may fear and demonise them. At the time of writing this book a 'hug a hoodie' campaign by a leading political party calls for more understanding of young people and of their behaviours, including crime and self-harm.

The Good Childhood Inquiry was commissioned by The Children's Society and launched in September 2006 as the UK's first independent national inquiry into childhood. Its aims were to renew society's understanding of modern childhood and to inform, improve and inspire our relationships with children. The report of the inquiry, *A Good Childhood*, is a collection of the evidence, recommendations and summaries of the themes discussed throughout the Inquiry (Children's Society 2009).

How does self-harm help young people?

Having discussed why young people may be more vulnerable to self-harm and how some experience highly stressful situations, we now look at the different ways in which they use self-harm. After all, given that so many young people self-harm, it must serve a function, even if that function is not fully understood.

For people who have not self-harmed or have not found themselves in a position where they considered self-harm as an option, the behaviour can be difficult to fathom. Many young people have voiced their opinions in clinical practice and on self-harm websites. Some have suggested that it is not possible to fully understand self-harm unless it has been directly experienced.

If we seek to understand why young people came to harm themselves in the first place, this may help us to develop preventative strategies and identify those at greatest risk.

> I feel so sad that I will now always be someone that has self-harmed. I wish I had told someone how I was feeling.
>
> Andrew, 15

Relief and release

Some young people stumble across self-harm by accident. For example, they cut themselves and either immediately feel better or later reflect on this as being helpful. They report feeling relieved and state that self-harm helps release tension. Consequently, they do it again at a later date and under similar circumstances. This is to feel the same sensation and reach the experience of feeling better again. It is therefore easy to see how a cycle of self-harm can evolve.

> I remember I couldn't believe what I'd just done – and how much better it made me feel.
>
> Kyle, 17

When self-harm involves physical pain, such as cutting and burning, young people often report that it reduces their emotional pain (Mental Health Foundation and Camelot Foundation 2006). At the time this can be an attractive option as the physical pain is often experienced as being more bearable than the emotional distress. Young people who have experienced some kind of trauma often report that self-harm becomes a temporary way to deal with their situation and associated feelings.

Communicating distress

On reflecting about their self-harm with professionals, many young people say how they wanted people to 'know' something. It was a way of communicating when they just could not find a way of putting things into words. This communication may relate to a particular trauma, for example a physical assault by someone at school, or be linked to a more pervasive problem in the family.

Often, young people don't know who to ask for help or even who they should ask. They may worry about putting more stress onto others. For example if a young person perceives that their parents are already stressed, they may be reluctant to burden them by talking about exam pressures.

For some young people who self-harm, triggers for the behaviour are clearly evident and self-harm is a way of coping in the absence of other healthier, safer alternatives. They may not be able to think clearly in a time of crisis and find it difficult to generate ideas about how to deal with the problem. They may believe that people around them do not care, will not understand, or do not have time to help or fail to take them seriously. These beliefs and perceptions may prevent young people from asking others for help in a situation where they are struggling to cope on their own.

Self-punishment and blame

One of the themes most commonly identified by young people for their self-harm, particularly for those that cut themselves, is the perceived need for punishment (Winchel and Stanley 1991; Favazza 1998; MacAniff and Kiselica 2001). As guidance from the NHS in Scotland points out, young people who cut themselves may be purging, or ridding themselves of poisons or 'dirty' feelings. Blood is a very visible sign of being alive, being punished and being ill. Some like the sight of their blood and may be soothed by its loss or seeing it washed away. The visual impact of cutting makes it a popular method of self-harm (NHS Scotland 2006).

The perceived need for punishment may be associated with past abuse, and self-harm can lead to trauma enactment which brings about the feelings a young person had when they were first traumatised. Self blame is also common. If a young person has struggled with problems for some time, their self-esteem may be very low. They may start to believe that some of the problems are directly their fault and conclude that they are to blame for everything.

> I use self-harm to punish and cleanse myself and to turn myself from blue to red. I am bad to the bone.

Some young people see themselves as dirty, often as a result of abuse. Self-harm may be a way of symbolically cleansing themselves of the contamination they feel. Negative beliefs can lead young people to develop a negative self-image. For some, this self-doubt evolves to the extent that they feel ugly, stupid or worthless. Such negative beliefs can lead to self-harm. For example, young people may cut themselves as punishment for being all the negative things they perceive themselves to be. Relief from feeling bad comes from the punishment that cutting provides.

> The badness I feel becomes unbearable. I can't take it any more so I cut. The relief is instant. It's like I've got what I deserve. The badness just drains away …

The young person with negative feelings is not helped by adults who overreact to their self-harming behaviour. Whilst it is normal for adults to sometimes feel shocked or upset when young people hurt themselves or place their lives at risk, expressing this to the young person is likely to make them feel further blamed and uncontained. Panicking and overreacting can be very frightening for the young person, and it is crucial to try and stay calm and take time to discuss with them what should be done next. If professionals are to provide effective support and be helpful, they must manage their own feelings and not add to the young person's distress. As difficult as it may sound, it is important to distance oneself from an excessive emotional reaction and be as supportive and understanding as possible.

Regaining control

For some people there are no clear triggers which precipitate their self-harm. Rather, they experience a gradual decline in mood and loss of emotional control. As they become increasingly despondent or distressed, their need to regain control increases. This change of mood state may relate to a specific mental health problem such as depression or labile emotions in general. Unexpected changes in mood and feelings and the subsequent need to regain control may also be associated with a history of or present experience of abuse. As well as feeling in control, young people report that self-harm can help to make them feel 'alive' again.

> I used to hurt myself so that I was in control and no one could hurt me more than I hurt myself.
>
> Curtis, 16

Regardless of the means by which a young person harms themselves, it is nonetheless an act of harm. Even though it may have served to prevent more serious damage or death, it still causes harm. Therefore, the objective of intervention with young people who are distressed or unhappy should always be to support them to cope in ways that do not cause harm. Whether self-harm becomes less commonly used as a way of coping is to some extent a public health priority. This is discussed further later in the book.

Emotional self-regulation

Self-regulation is the ability to manage and control one's emotions. As a child, regulation is provided by parents and carers through the process of attachment and the provision of a secure base. Experiences such as discipline and boundaries, rewards, punishments and limit setting enable children to internalise the ability to regulate. Over time, most young people develop the skills of self-regulation. These include self-soothing and self-distracting techniques to avoid aversive experiences, and the ability to talk with others and negotiate ways to resolve difficulties and challenges.

Many young people who self-harm report that they find it difficult to control their emotions, and these testimonials are supported in the research literature (Miller *et al.* 2007). They describe having problems managing their anger or sadness and report feeling overwhelmed when upset or challenged. Self-harm becomes a way of coping with strong feelings young people struggle to regulate in non-destructive ways.

Dissociation

Dissociation is a trauma-based condition. It is a way of separating, as a protective strategy, from something unbearable. Dissociation is described as being on a continuum. From being associated, young people temporarily switch off, blank out, and cut off from the body. This process involves a splitting off from oneself to develop an alternative self (Spandler and Warner 2007). Dissociative processes often underpin self-harming behaviour, such as cutting or burning. As Sellen (2008) points out, if a young person has a history in which they have learnt to manage strong sensations through self-harm, it is not surprising that they will feel a sense of relief, even comfort, from dissociation.

Some people who experience dissociation and self-harm as a means of feeling in touch with themselves. Self-harm makes them feel real or alive again. For young people who are further down the dissociation continuum, the risks are greater as the capacity for self-control diminishes. Young people sometimes report feeling frightened about what has happened while they were in this dissociated state. During times of dissociation, young people may not be able to describe what has happened. They may be vague about the circumstances and their feelings and imply that they did not feel present when the self-harm occurred. In order to reduce the risk of repetition of self-harm, young people need therapeutic help to understand and manage dissociation.

Habitual self-harm

For some young people, several of the benefits they report about self-harm act as positive reinforcers. The act of self-harm temporarily makes them feel better and the behaviour can evolve to become habitual. Like many habits, some young people may find it more difficult than others to refrain or stop what may become increasingly problematic.

> When I was self-harming numerous times a day, I think I became addicted to the feeling of harming more than anything else.

It may be helpful to think about how self-harm compares to other habits or addictions. Smoking cigarettes, drinking alcohol or overeating are all things people develop gradually. Some people do them more than others, and for many they reduce over time without significant effort or professional help. For others, they make a decision and stop suddenly, never to do it again or relapse every now and again. They experience regular cravings and after indulging, get a sense of relief. Some do not manage to stop these habits which can eventually become harmful or even fatal. In some ways, self-harm is no different and the way in which each young person develops their self-harming behaviour is different.

Suicidal intent

The vast majority of young people use self-harm as a coping strategy, as a way to survive and deal with the emotional distress they are experiencing. However, it is important to note again that only a minority of young people harm themselves with the intention of killing themselves. Determining suicidal intent is often a challenging task which is discussed further in Chapters 6 and 7.

Why do some young people stop self-harming?

Just as it is crucial to seek explanations for why young people self-harm, understanding what makes them reduce or stop is also important. There is a lack of peer-reviewed research exploring the reasons why people stop self-harming, and the little research that has been done focuses on adults (Sinclair and Green 2005). The Centre for Suicide Research has an online resource that summarises and catalogues studies undertaken by the department on self-harm and suicide. Looking at the general trends and statistics over the past 30 years, incidents of self-harm tend to peek in the late teens and show a decline with age, though this pattern does vary according to gender.

Some young people therefore appear to grow out of their self-harming behaviour. They may be assisted to replace self-harm with alternative coping strategies, or find ways to stop without professional help. Others stop as they begin to appraise their problems differently and acquire more independence and power to change their lives. Consequently, their problems or difficulties are reduced or cease altogether. As young people grow older they may come to develop a more positive view of themselves, believe that they have a choice and conclude that self-harm does not have to be part of their lives.

Again, for some young people this process can occur without professional help, whereas for others they require support to develop self-esteem and the skills to cope in the face of stress and adversity. Some young people go on to help others, either virtually or in person, or by working for organisations such as Harmless. This is a user-led organisation that provides a range of services related to self-harm, including support, information, training and consultancy to people who self-harm, their friends and families and professionals.

Whereas many young people reduce their self-harm gradually, others suddenly make a decision to stop and do so quite quickly. We have heard that some people view their self-harm as a habit that can be very difficult to stop, even when they are trying hard to do so. Reducing or stopping self-harm can be understood in the same way someone might try to stop smoking cigarettes.

Scarring

Some young people who have cut or burnt themselves come to terms with their self-harm. They accept their scars as being part of them and regard them as part of what happened at a particular time in their life. They may have been unaware of the permanent damage that would be caused, or chose not to consider the longer term consequences of their actions.

> I used to be really embarrassed and hide my scars by wearing long sleeves in summer, but now I wear short sleeves if its nice. I don't care what people think anymore.

Others are aware that their self-harming behaviour may have more permanent consequences, or they do not want to be visibly reminded of painful times. It is often this foresight that can act as a strong motivator for young people to find alternative ways to cope and either reduce or stop their self-harming. Many young people are concerned about their body image, how they look and how others see them. Consequently, they are keen to find non-destructive ways to manage their problems and difficulties. However, rather than stop cutting as a result of concerns about body image, some young people harm themselves in less visible places, such as their thighs and stomach. Additionally, self-harm which is less visible attracts less concern, interest or disapproval from family, friends or adults who are concerned about their welfare.

Media reporting

We have read that popular media plays a key role in shaping views, attitudes and social norms. Even if young people have no direct experience of someone who has self-harmed, they often relate to characters on TV or in the music industry that are associated with self-harm. Indeed, various producers of soap operas, artists and musicians have been criticised for increasing self-harm and suicide in young people (Armstrong 2006). Young people who are depressed or who have made a previous suicide attempt themselves may be particularly affected in an adverse way (Cheng *et al.* 2007a and b).

Phillips (1982) demonstrated an increase in suicide up to ten days after television news reports about someone killing themselves. Improving media reporting was identified as one of the six priority areas in the National Suicide Prevention Strategy for England in 2002. In 2006, newspaper editors were urged to discourage reporting in depth about self-harm and suicide, and the Samaritans have since produced comprehensive media guidelines for the sensitive reporting of suicide and self-harm (Samaritans 2008). The Editor's Code also includes a requirement in relation to self-harm and suicide. This states that in cases involving grief and shock, enquiries must be carried out and approaches made with sympathy and discretion.

Due to the risks of imitation described earlier, when reporting suicides, the Code states that care should be taken to avoid excessive detail about the methods used (Press Complaints Commission Code of Practice). The National CAMHS Review (Department for Children, Schools and Families 2008a) has also called on the press to consider more carefully their responsibilities when reporting on stories of suicide and self-harm.

Despite guidance, concerns about the reporting of suicides continue. Following a spate of suicides by young people in Bridgend Wales in 2009, global newspaper and television interest was attracted by a media release of what Garthwaite (2009) called 'sensational, provocative and inaccurate statements'. This caused distress to the families and friends of those who had died, heightened anxiety of young people in schools and gave unhelpful messages about self-harm to the public. Generalisations based on small figures always require close scrutiny, and terms such as 'suicide epidemic' are often unhelpful and misleading.

Following the Bridgend suicides, huge resources were put in place to provide support to the community. This was partly because people bereaved by suicide are themselves at increased risk of suicide and self-harm (Brent *et al.* 1996), and because it is also known that one suicide may lead to others within a limited period of time and geographical area (Brent *et al.* 1989; Gould *et al.* 1990).

It is not only in the UK that negative media reporting can increase suicide rates among the vulnerable. A study in Hong Kong reported that following the death of a famous pop singer who died after jumping from a height, there was a significant increase in suicide in the general public, many of whom also died by jumping (Yip *et al.* 2006). Interestingly, following the death of US singer Kurt Cobain, who shot himself in 1994, an increase in suicide among young people was not noted. Various reasons for this have been proposed for this including positive media reporting. There was also the suggestion that the substantial efforts made by Kurt Cobain's widow, Courtney Love, to present his suicide in a negative fashion may have counteracted any potential glamorisation of his death (Gould 2001).

Various guidelines suggest that responsible reporting of suicide should not include speculation about motives and circumstances, but come from a position of compassion and social responsibility (Gunnell 1994; WHO 2000b). Whilst journalists are under pressure to file reports that are of the moment and in the public interest, there remains the responsibility not to glamorise the story or intrude on the grief and shock of those affected (Samaritans 2008).

Summary

The reasons young people self-harm are widespread and often complex. However, consistent themes emerge from research and from what young people tell us themselves. There has been extensive international research that has addressed the association between self-harm and stressful life events, drug and alcohol use, child abuse and neglect, domestic violence and mental disorder. It is not always possible to solve the problems that the young person identifies as being stressful. However, the objective should be about helping them to manage the problem more effectively. This can be the underlying issues or the actual self-harm itself.

If we are serious about reducing self-harm in young people, then there are several areas to address. First, we need more knowledge and understanding about adolescent and young adult development. There is a growing awareness that prevention of childhood difficulties and early intervention by universal services is likely to produce better outcomes than intervention in adolescence or adulthood. Parents are often supported by child development centres, health and maternity services, nurseries, family centres, and numerous community resources. The same diversity of facilities and supports does not currently exist to guide young people and parents or carers through the rocky terrain of adolescence.

Second, we need to broaden our approaches to engage young people and increase access to support for young people who want it. Increasingly, young people are using social networking and electronic messaging to communicate about self-harm. The real scale of the effects of virtual relationships is not known and needs to be explored, and perhaps more appropriately vetted. The proliferation of self-harm blogs, message boards and websites may be a mixed blessing. Further research and monitoring is needed in this area.

Third, we need to continue to develop and offer young people a variety of services to help meet their individual needs. Finally, as professionals we must take responsibility for checking our own beliefs and perceptions about self-harm. We must endeavour not to make unhelpful judgements about young people who self-harm, and instead offer them support, understanding and compassion. Finally, we must remain serious about reducing stigma. Despite professional guidelines and public campaigns about mental health and self-harm, discrimination continues. This adversely affects outcomes for children and young people and society as a whole.

3 What works for young people who self-harm?

Key points:

- The evaluation and treatment of adolescent self-harm and suicide is an under-researched area of work both in the UK and the USA. A number of studies have been conducted to investigate epidemiological factors and risk indicators, but there is much less robust evidence about treatments that are known to be effective.
- Drawing firm conclusions about the effectiveness of interventions for young people who self-harm is problematic. The ability to devise effective interventions is significantly compromised by limited knowledge of the natural course following a self-harm or suicide attempt.
- Young people who repeat self-harm are very often more disturbed and often experience greater psychosocial adversity and coexisting problems than those who harm themselves once. The risk of repetition is greater in the first few weeks following self-harm, and repetition increases the risk of eventual suicide.
- NICE has produced guidelines on the short-term physical and psychological management and secondary prevention of self-harm in primary and secondary care. The guidelines bring together the evidence for self-harm interventions and set good practice guidelines for professionals and organisations that provide services for people who self-harm.
- Despite a range of guidance, many people do not know how to respond effectively to young people who self-harm, and what works and does not work is not common knowledge.

Introduction

Earlier chapters reviewed some of the literature about young people who self-harm, those who attempt suicide and young people who kill themselves. This is helpful in generating important insights and clues about the kind of risks and epidemiological factors which surround the issue. This chapter focuses on the evaluation and treatment of young people who self-harm. Aftercare following acts of self-harm by young people is an under-researched area of study in the UK (Black 1992). Much of the literature examining short- and long-term outcomes has focused on adult self-harm and is mainly classified as attempted suicide regardless of intent. This is a major public health concern which will be discussed further in Chapter 10.

Gunnell and Frankel (1994) suggested that drawing conclusions about the effectiveness of interventions for young people who self-harm is an area of controversy. The ability to devise effective interventions for adolescent self-harm is significantly compromised by limited knowledge of the natural course following a suicide attempt (Spirito *et al.* 1989). Therefore, before we consider treatment options for young people who self-harm, we must review what is known about the outcomes for this population.

Evaluating outcomes

There are several factors which impact on the evaluation of outcomes for young people who harm themselves. These present numerous challenges and difficulties for researchers and clinicians. First, statistical information on attempted suicides has historically been unreliable and biased. Much of the literature has suggested that the number of attempted suicides is grossly under-reported, (US Department of Health and Human Services 1981), and the true incidence of non-fatal self-harm is not known. This is likely to be because many young people do not receive medical treatment following their attempt.

Second, when reporting self-harm, researchers and clinicians vary widely in their definitions of suicidal behaviour, as discussed in Chapter 2. Failure to agree a common definition of what we mean by self-harm presents difficulties in data collection and analysis. Diagnostic criteria vary considerably, and there is a notable lack of agreement in relation to contributing factors. In their Oxford study, Hawton *et al.* (1982) used a simple classification scheme which focused primarily on behaviour rather than psychiatric symptoms (see Table 3.1).

Data was collected on the three groups shown in Table 3.1 and marked differences were evident. The difficulties experienced by Group one focused almost exclusively on current relationships, whereas the problems experienced by young people in Group two and three were more complex. As Table 3.2 shows, the group with chronic problems and behaviour disturbance had many

Table 3.1 Classification of self-harm (adapted from Hawton *et al.* 1982)

Group one	Acute	Young people have problems which have lasted for less than one month and there is an absence of behavioural disturbance.
Group two	Chronic	Young people have problems which have lasted for more than one month and there is an absence of behavioural disturbance.
Group three	Chronic with behavioural disturbance	Young people have had problems which have lasted for one month or more and there are also behavioural problems.

Table 3.2 Characteristics of adolescent self-poisoners categorised according to a simple classification scheme (adapted from Hawton *et al.* 1982)

	Group one Acute	Group two Chronic	Group three Chronic with behavioural disturbance
Broken homes		+	+ + +
Family history of mental health problems			+ + +
Poor relationship with mother		+	+ + +
Poor relationship with father	+	+ +	+ + +
Previous mental health problems or treatment		+	+ + +
Previous overdose/self-harm			+ +
Number of problems	+	+ +	+ + +
Psychiatric symptoms		+	+ + +

Note: + indicates which characteristic is displayed by members of each group.

more problems. When assessing outcomes it is unclear as to what extent findings can be generalised due to such discrepancies.

A further difficulty with interpreting outcome research is that many studies fail to give an adequate age distribution and the samples often include older adolescents and the adult population. This provides greater numbers and has fewer methodological considerations, but there are likely to be major differences between this group and a group of much younger adolescents. Therefore, the results of many studies cannot be generalised adequately to children and adolescents.

Third, some young people may reject offers of help with their self-harm and this may affect the outcomes for such young people. It is likely that they will present in crisis, and initial appeals for help are made closer to home, for example through teachers and friends. Following admission to an accident and emergency department, their first priority may be to get out of hospital rather than exploring treatment options. Some young people presenting to emergency departments receive no further treatment. Berman and Caroll (1984) believe that the psychopathology of parents affects the young person receiving appropriate treatment and follow-up. Some families prefer to forget the whole incident. Data suggests that approximately half of all self-harmers do not receive any formal psychotherapy (Keinhorst *et al.* 1987).

Knowledge of psychological status of adolescents who self-harm and those who attempt suicide is confounded by the heterogeneity of the population. Hawton *et al.* (1982) looked at outcomes in terms of overall adjustment using the classification schema referred to above. The 50 adolescents who had self-poisoned in the Oxford study were interviewed one month after their overdoses. Due to the relatively short follow-up period, there was an unusually high follow-up rate. The outcome was that 66 per cent had improved,

32 per cent remained unchanged and 2 per cent reported feeling worse. Overall adjustment, using the classification scheme shown in Table 3.3, demonstrated a clear difference between the three groups.

Ninety per cent of subjects in the acute group were rated as improved whereas 75 per cent in the chronic group and only 25 per cent in the chronic group with behaviour disturbance admitted to overall improvement. It is evident that short-term outcomes are relatively good whereas young people in the chronic with behavioural disturbances group had more long-term difficulties. Spirito *et al.* (1989) suggested that many adolescent suicide attempters experience continued disturbances after their acute episode.

Repetition of self-harm

Young people who repeatedly self-harm present greater concern because of their psychological co-morbidity and the increased risk of suicide. When evaluating outcomes, repetition rates are an important area to be investigated. Young people who repeat self-harm are very often more disturbed and often experience greater psychosocial difficulties and coexisting problems. Kreitman and Casey (1988) noted that young people who repeatedly harm themselves are high consumers of health service resources.

Follow-up studies of suicide attempts by young people have suggested that approximately one in ten will make a further suicide attempt during the year after their first attempt. A large study of self-harm repetition by nearly 2,500 young people aged 12–20 demonstrated that 6.3 per cent harmed themselves within one year of their initial admission (Goldacre and Hawton 1988). However, these statistics were only an approximation and likely to be an underestimate as the numbers were based on hospital admissions. More recent studies suggest that up to a quarter of young people repeat self-harm within a year of

Table 3.3 Short-term outcome and repetition of attempts in 50 adolescent self-poisoners (adapted from Hawton *et al.* 1982, Oxford study)

Group self-classification*	Improved overall adjustment one month after the overdose	Repeat attempts in year after the overdose
Acute (Group 1) (n=10)	90% (n=9)	10% (n=1)
Chronic (Group 2) (n=28)	75% (n=21)	0% (n=0)
Chronic with behavioural disturbance (Group 3) (n=12)	25% ** (n=3)	50% *** (n=6)

* see table for definition of the self-classification schema used

** χ^2 = 12.57 (Group 3 versus Groups 1+2) p <0.01

*** χ^2 = 13.29 (Group 3 versus Groups 1+2) p <0.001

an earlier episode (Sakinofsky 2000; Owens *et al.* 2002). The risk of repetition is greater in the first few weeks following self-harm and repetition increases the risk of eventual suicide (Zahl and Hawton 2004).

Whilst this is clearly important in terms of risk assessment and prevention of repetition, identification of high risk periods following the initial act of self-harm have received little attention in research. In another study of repeat self-harm, data from the first episode of self-harm were re-examined. Young people who were repeat self-harmers compared to those who had harmed themselves only once were more likely to be experiencing ongoing life stresses, difficulties in school and more serious suicidal intent (Gispert *et al.* 1987). Repetition measures to assess risk in adults who self-harm have been published. However, similar measures for use with children and adolescents have yet to be developed.

Brent (1997) provides an overview related to the aftercare of self-harm. He was particularly concerned with the suicidal risk and environmental factors most likely to maintain self-harming behaviour. Brent identified important key elements, such as obtaining a 'no suicide' contract, addressing non-compliance, family education, remediation of social skills, and problem solving deficits, alongside the treatment of coexisting psychiatric disorders.

Adverse psychiatric and psychosocial outcomes

In addition to repetition, suicide attempts have been associated with other outcomes, such as difficulties with social and psychological adjustment. Pfeffer *et al.* (1991) carried out a six- to eight-year comparative study of 100 pre-adolescent and adolescent inpatients in New York. The strongest risk factor for a repeat suicide attempt was the presence of a mood disorder. Pfeffer *et al.* (1993) also found that girls were more likely than boys to make multiple suicide attempts during the six- to eight-year follow-up. The evidence demonstrated that many of the repeat suicide attempts occurred among young people who reported a suicide attempt at the time of initial assessment. Half of this group reported multiple suicide attempts during the follow-up period. Asarow *et al.* (1987) found that inability to access social support from significant individuals and minimal social activities with peers were risk factors for continued suicidal acts.

In Pfeffer's follow-up study (1993) investigating rates and psychosocial risk factors for suicide attempts during follow-up, it was observed that children who attempted suicide in the follow-up period were 3.5 times more likely to have a mood disorder a year after their initial attempt. Other reports indicate that even when mood disorder resolves, problems with social adjustment can persist. Lewinsohn *et al.* (1994) found that outcomes of childhood self-harm were similar to that of depression.

Pfeffer and colleagues (1993) also found that repetition of self-harm is often linked to episodes of depression. However, Kerfoot *et al.* (1996) suggested that major depressive disorder often remits following acts of self-harm. Pfeffer (1993) reported that young people who harmed themselves or had suicidal ideas were more likely to have a variety of psychiatric disorders and poorer social adjustment during the post-attempt course. The findings from this study suggest a chronic morbidity as these children grow up. Pfeffer *et al.* (1993) concluded that these children required a multi-modal approach, geared towards reducing rates of repeat self-harm and the most fatal outcome of all, completed suicide.

Completed suicide

One of the longer follow-up studies is a 10- to 15-year follow-up study of over 1,500 patients using registers from Swedish institutions (Otto 1972). The study found that 67 people died, with 80 per cent by suicide. Granboulan *et al.* (1995) found that out of a sample of 265 hospitalised adolescents, 15 subjects had died within a follow-up period of nine years. One died from natural causes, five had committed suicide and nine had died from unnatural or violent causes other than suicide. In all 14 cases, the cause of death appeared to be linked to disorders which first started during adolescence. It is widely recognised that official suicide rates conceal the real scale of fatalities, particularly with the younger population.

Recent research has noted the rising rates of completed suicide as part of a wider trend of increases in a range of psychosocial disorders. WHO (2004) estimated that about 1.5 million people die by suicide each year. Again, this is an estimate and the true figure may be considerably higher. It has been suggested that the actual numerical burden and years of life lost to suicide may be greater in young people (Jamison and Hawton 2005).

Assessing outcomes – randomised controlled trials

The findings reviewed thus far suggest that young people who harm themselves are at risk of a range of adverse outcomes. How can these outcomes best be prevented? Randomised controlled trials (RCTs) are seen as the 'gold standard' in the world of research. They are used to objectively test the efficacy of treatments, and randomisation is used to balance confounding factors between treatment groups. Additionally, there has been extensive work conducted using qualitative techniques and invaluable personal testimonies which could be the subject of a book in itself. However, the extent of the available RCT research literature precludes the need to include these other informative, well conducted studies in this chapter.

A key review of RCTs was conducted by Hawton *et al.* (1998b), who carried out a systematic review identifying and analysing the findings from all RCTs which had examined the efficacy of treatments on patients of all ages who had self-harmed. A total of 20 trials were identified in this review and were classified into ten categories according to type of treatment received – e.g. problem solving therapy versus standard aftercare. The review included studies in which experimental subjects were offered some form of problem solving therapy, compared with the standard or routine care (treatment as usual) received in the control group. The studies are summarised in Table 3.4. Rates of repetition were measured as opposed to actual suicides owing to the large numbers which would be required to evaluate trials in terms of completed suicide. The quality of concealment from allocation was rated in each study, with 1 indicating poor quality, 2 medium quality, and 3 high quality.

The results of the systematic review indicated that there is insufficient evidence to make strong recommendations about the type of aftercare needed to prevent recurrence of self-harm. Treatment options are likely to vary greatly between different countries and regions. One of the limitations not highlighted was the vast difference in the age between the populations studied. Some children were as young as 12 and other people were as old as 68. This provides extreme heterogeneity between subjects, and ultimately causes difficulties in designing appropriate treatment packages.

Randomised controlled trials with adolescents who self-harm

In a book about children and young people, it is pertinent to identify those RCTs which have investigated outcomes with adolescents who self-harm. A review of published literature revealed only six relevant RCTs, one of which (Cotgrove *et al.* 1995) was highlighted in Hawton's systematic review (Hawton *et al.* 1998b).

Cotgrove and colleagues (1995) conducted a study where adolescents discharged from hospital following a suicide attempt were randomly allocated to two arms of a trial. The first group received standard care, plus a token (green card) which allowed them to be readmitted to hospital on demand. The second group (control group) received just the standard management. The hypothesis behind the study was that in order to reduce future self-harm, the young person could use their green card to temporarily 'escape' from their environment until the crisis or stressful situation had resolved. Follow-up was at one year and involved a total of 105 participants. All the young people were aged 16 or under with a mean age of 14.9 years. Forty-five per cent received the green card treatment and 55 per cent were allocated to the control group.

The comparison revealed that six per cent in the treatment group made further suicide attempts (11 per cent making use of their green card), whereas in the control group 12 per cent made a further suicide attempt. The other interesting finding was that the clinician's crude estimate of risk from the index episode (low, medium, high) correlated significantly with repeated self-harm or suicide attempts. Cotgrove *et al.* (1995) reported that the young people used their green cards appropriately and concluded that this very simple technique had a lot of potential to researchers and clinicians in the field.

A second randomised controlled trial with adolescents was of a home-based family intervention for children who had poisoned themselves. Harrington *et al.* (1998a) compared a brief home-based programme conducted by child psychiatric social workers with adolescents and their families, plus routine

Table 3.4 Summary of participants, interventions, follow-up period, size of trial and quality of concealment of allocation (from Hawton *et al.* 1998)

Study (Country)	Details of participants	Interventions	No. randomised (no. lost to follow-up or excluded)	Follow-up period (months)	Quality of concealment of allocation
		Problem solving therapy versus standard aftercare			
Gibbons *et al.* 1978 (UK)	Patients over 17 years who presented to A&E department. After deliberate self-poisoning: Repeaters and first timers: 71% female	Experimental (n=200): crisis orientated, time limited, task centred social work at home (problem solving intervention). Control (n=200): routine service – 54% GP referral, 33% psychiatric referral, 13 % other referral	400	12	3
Hawton *et al.* 1987 (UK)	Patients over 16 years admitted to general hospital for self-poisoning: 31 % repeaters: 66% female	Experimental (n=41): outpatient problem orientated therapy by non-medical clinicians. Control (n=39): GP care (for example, individual support, marital therapy) after advice from clinician	80	12	3
Salkovskis *et al.* 1990 (UK)	Patients aged 16–65 (mean 27.5) referred by duty psychiatrist after antidepressant self-poisoning; assessed in A&E department; all repeaters with high risk of further repetition: 50% female	Experimental (n=12): domiciliary cognitive behavioural problem solving treatment. Control (n=8): treatment as usual (GP care)	20	12	3
McLeavey et al. 1994 (Ireland)	Patients aged 15–45 (mean 24.4) admitted to A&E department after self-poisoning: 35.6% repeaters: 74% female	Experimental (n=19): interpersonal problem solving skills training. Control (n=2): brief problem solving therapy	39	12	1

continued overleaf

Intensive care plus outreach versus standard care

Chowdhury et al. 1973 (UK)	Patients (all repeaters) admitted to general hospital after deliberate self-harm: 57% female	Experimental (n=71): special aftercare – regular outpatient appointments: patients also seen without appointments: home visits to patients who missed appointments: emergency 24-hour telephone access. Control (n=84): normal aftercare – patient appointments with psychiatrist and/or social worker: non-attendees not pursued	155	6	1
Welu 1977 (USA)	Suicide attempters over 16 years brought to A&E department: 60% repeaters: % female not given	Experimental (n=63): special outreach programme – community mental health team contacted patient immediately after discharge: home visit arranged: weekly/ twice weekly contact with therapist. Control (n=57): routine care – appointment for evaluation at the community mental health centre next day at request of treating physician	120 (1)	4	1
Hawton et al. 1981 (UK)	Patients ≥ 16 years (mean 25.3) admitted to general hospital after deliberate self-poisoning; 32 % repeaters: 70% female	Experimental (n=48): domiciliary therapy (brief problem orientated) as often as therapist thought necessary: open telephone access to general hospital service. Control (n=48): outpatient therapy once a week in outpatient clinic in general hospital	96	12	3
Allard et al. 1992 (Canada)	Patients seen in A&E department for suicide attempts: 50% repeaters: 55% female	Experimental (n=76): intensive intervention – schedule of visits was arranged including at least one home visit; therapy provided when needed: reminders (telephone or written) and home visits made if appointments missed. Control (n=74): treatment by another staff team in the same hospital	150 (24)	12	3

Table 3.4 continued

Study (Country)	Details of participants	Interventions	No. randomised (no. lost to follow-up or excluded)	Follow-up period	Quality of concealment of allocation
		Intensive care plus outreach versus standard care			
Van Heeringen et al. 1995 (Belgium)	Patients seen ≥ 15 years treated in A&E department after suicide attempt: 30% repeaters: 43% female	Experimental (n=258): special care – home visits by nurse to patients who did not keep outpatient appointments, reasons for not attending discussed and patient encouraged to attend. Control (n=258): outpatient appointments only: non-compliant patients not visited	516 (125)	12	3
Van de Sande et al. 1997 (Netherlands)	Patients ≥ 16 years (mean 36.3) admitted to hospital after suicide attempt: 73% repeaters: 66%	Experimental (n = 140): brief psychiatric unit admission, encouraging patients to contact unit on discharge: outpatient therapy plus 24-hour emergency access to unit. Control (n=134): usual care – 25% admitted to hospital, 65% outpatient referral	274	12	3
		Emergency card versus standard aftercare			
Morgan et al. 1993 (UK)	Mean age 30 years: patients admitted after first episode of deliberate self-harm: % female not given	Experimental (n=101): standard care plus green card (emergency card indicating that doctor was available and how to contact them). Control (n=111): standard care – for example, referral back to primary health care team, psychiatric inpatient admission	112	12	3
Cotgrove et al. 1995 (UK)	Patients aged 12.2–16.7 (mean 14.9) admitted after deliberate self-harm: % repeaters not given: 85% female	Experimental (n=47): standard care plus green card (emergency card) – green card acted as passport to readmission into paediatric ward in local hospital. Control (n=58): standard follow-up treatment from clinic or child psychiatry department	105	12	1

continued overleaf

Study	Patients	Intervention			
Dialectical behaviour therapy versus standard aftercare					
Linehan *et al.* 1991 (USA)	Patients aged 18–45 who had self-harmed within eight weeks before entering study: all female all multiple repeaters of self-harm	Experimental (n=32) dialectical behaviour therapy (individual and group work) for one year: telephone access to therapist. Control (n=31): treatment as usual: 73% individual psychotherapy	63 (24)	12	3
Inpatient behaviour therapy versus inpatient insight orientated therapy					
Liberman and Eckman 1981 (USA)	Patients (mean (range) age 29.7 (18–47)) all repeaters: patients referred by psychiatric emergency service or hospital A&E department after deliberate self-harm: 67% female	Experimental (n=12) inpatient treatment with behaviour therapy. Control (n=12): inpatient treatment with insight orientated therapy: both groups received individual and group therapy plus aftercare at community mental health centre or with private therapist	24	24	2
Same therapist (continuity of care) versus different therapist (change of care)					
Torhorst *et al.* 1987 (Germany)	Patients referred to toxological department of Technical University Munich after deliberate self-poisoning: 48% repeaters: 62% female	Experimental (n=68): continuity of care – therapy with same therapist who assessed patient in hospital after attempt. Control (n=73): change of care – therapy with different therapist than seen at hospital assessment	141 (8)	12	2
General hospital admission versus discharge					
Waterhouse and Platt 1990 (UK)	Patients ≥ 16 years (mean 30.3) admitted to A&E department for deliberate self-harm: 36% repeaters: 63% female	Experimental (n=38): general hospital admission. Control (n=39): discharge from hospital: on discharge both groups advised to contact GP if they needed further help	77	16	3

Table 3.4 continued

Study (Country)	Details of participants	Interventions	No. randomised (no. lost to follow-up or excluded)	Follow-up period	Quality of concealment of allocation
		Flupenthixol versus placebo			
Montgomery et al. 1979 (UK)	Patients aged 16–68 (mean 35.3) admitted after suicidal act: all repeaters: 70% female	Experimental (n=18): 20 mg intramuscular flupenthixol decanoate for six months. Control (n=19) placebo for six months	37 (7)	6	3
		Long-term therapy versus short-term therapy			
Torhorst et al. 1988 (Germany)	All patients repeaters who had deliberately self-poisoned; % female not given	Experimental (n=40): long-term therapy – one therapy session a month for 12 months. Control (n=40) short-term therapy – 12 weekly therapy sessions for three months: all participants had brief crisis intervention (three days) in hospital	114	3	3
		Antidepressants versus placebo			
Hirsch et al. 1982 R Draper, S Hirsch (quoted by Hawton et al. 1998) (UK)	Patients aged 16–65 admitted after deliberate self-poisoning; % repeaters and % female not given	Experimental (n=76): antidepressants – either 30–60 mg mianserin for six weeks or 75–150 mg nomifensine for six weeks. Control (n=38): placebo for six weeks	114	3	3
Montgomery et al. 1983 (UK)	Patients with personality disorders mean age 35.7) admitted to medical ward after deliberate self-harm: all repeaters: 66% female	Experimental (n=17): mianserin 30 mg for six months. Control (n=21): placebo	38	6	3

care with subjects who received routine care only. The hypothesis was that the new treatment would lead to lower levels of suicidal ideation and that the families would be able to function better as a whole. Repetition was not included as the main outcome measure, although data was presented on rates of repetition. In total, 85 young people were allocated to the treatment group and 77 to the control group.

Overall, the findings demonstrated no greater effect of treatment than offered by routine care. However with a non-depressed subgroup, those having the family intervention had significantly lower levels of suicidal thinking than those who did not. The authors considered whether there seemed to be an effect of treatment with young people who did not have a depressive disorder. Brent and colleagues (1997) reported a similar trend. They concluded that other interventions, such as individual therapy and cognitive behaviour therapy (CBT) approaches may be more effective with young people who take overdoses.

In a further randomised controlled trial, Wood *et al.* (2001) investigated the benefits for adolescents randomised to either a group treatment referred to as 'developmental group psychotherapy' plus usual care (DGP) or treatment as usual (TAU). Sixty-three young people were recruited to either arm of the trial. The young people were followed up on average seven months after entry into the trial. Adolescents who received the group treatment demonstrated a significant reduction in self-harming behaviour (six per cent in the DGP group versus 32 per cent in the TAU group at seven months' follow-up). The young people in the group programme had fewer episodes overall, and those who repeated their self-harm had a longer time to the first repetition in the active treatment group (7 weeks in the DGP group versus 11 weeks in the TAU group). However, there were no differences in suicidal thinking or depression scores.

On the strength of this study by Wood *et al.* (2001), and to test the efficacy of the intervention in other locations, the same team commenced a large multi-centred trial. Internationally, this is currently the largest trial of young people who repeatedly self-harm. In total, 366 young people aged between 12 and 17 were recruited across eight different sites, involving eight specialised Child and Adolescent Mental Health Services (CAMHS) teams. The trial was a two-arm, single blinded, randomised allocation trial of the manualised group treatment (DGP) in addition to usual care, compared to usual care alone. Primary outcome assessment was similar to the previous trial, but also included an economic evaluation and, perhaps controversially, an adapted version of the Structured Clinical Interview for *DSM-IV* axis II personality disorders (SCID-II) which is used with adults. The results of this important RCT are currently being analysed, and the final report will be published in summer 2010 (Green *et al.* 2010).

Bennewith *et al.* (2002) evaluated a general practice-based intervention whereby GPs were given management guidelines for good practice involving self-harm, and subsequently proactively offered clients with self-harming behaviour the opportunity for a consultation. Although the study was a particularly well conducted RCT with a large sample size (n=1,932), it failed to find any significant differences between the intervention and non-intervention groups on any of the three outcome measures that were evaluated (repeat episodes of self-harm; number of repeat episodes; and time to first repetition). This rather disappointing outcome is unfortunately supported by the broader range of general practice-based training and other initiatives evaluated in the wider literature.

A further RCT by Carter and colleagues (2005) evaluated ongoing contact via postcards sent to people following discharge from hospital following self-poisoning, the most common form of self-harm by young people. The results were slightly more optimistic, but still produced limited positive outcomes. No significant differences were found in the absolute likelihood of further admissions. However, the intervention group – who received eight supportive postcards enquiring about their well-being over a 12-month period – showed a substantive and significant reduction in the total number of episodes recorded. For the control group, 192 episodes were recorded versus 101 for the intervention group. For a very minimalist intervention this is quite a substantial outcome in clinical terms. Further evaluation of the Carter study demonstrated that the impact primarily related to improvements for women rather than men, suggesting that the intervention may benefit from targeted rather than general implementation.

Finally, a quantitative self-harm study by Kapur *et al.* (2004a) involved a retrospective cohort study of people attending A&E departments following self-poisoning. Following adjustment for baseline differences, receiving a psychosocial assessment was not found to be associated with reduced repetition rates. However, being referred for specialist follow-up did reduce rates of subsequent repetition. This was a particularly well conducted study with a large sample size (n=658).

Systematic reviews

Systematic reviews seek to identify, appraise and evaluate all high quality research evidence in a particular area. An overview of systematic reviews conducted by the Scottish Executive (2008) identified seven published reviews involving adolescents and young people and these are summarised in Table 3.5 below. Overall, these studies conclude that some treatments may show promise, but more research is needed to provide adequate evidence.

Other studies

The review of the effectiveness of interventions to prevent suicide and suicidal behaviour (Scottish Executive 2008) did not identify many high quality studies. In addition to the RCTs identified in Table 3.5, the review noted only two other studies which were considered to be well conducted.

In the first study, Perseius *et al.* (2003) looked at outcomes in the context of both self-harm and suicide attempts, with dialectical behaviour therapy

Table 3.5 Systematic reviews of interventions to prevent self-harm and suicide in young people (from Scottish Executive 2008)

Authors	Outline of review	Conclusion
Hepp *et al.* (2004) (25 RCTs)	Psychological and psychosocial interventions involving people who had attempted suicide or engaged in deliberate self-harm	Minimal interventions (e.g. green card initiatives) and psychodynamic interventions (e.g. CBT and DBT) show promise but more research is needed to provide adequate evidence
Macgowan (2004) (10 RCTs)	Psychosocial treatments in adolescents	A number of treatments are cited as promising, but the authors conclude that current evidence of efficacy is weak and research designs are poor
Merry *et al.* (2004) (13 RCTs)	Psychological and/or psycho-educational interventions involving children and adolescents	There is insufficient evidence to warrant the introduction of depression prevention programmes to reduce suicide attempts and completed suicide
Ploeg *et al.* (1996) (11 RCTs)	Curriculum-based prevention programmes with adolescents involving prospective studies with a control group or before/after evaluation	There is currently insufficient evidence to support curriculum-based prevention programmes. The evidence suggests there may be both beneficial and harmful effects on attitudes related to suicide
Gould *et al.* (2003)	Psychological and pharmacological treatments with people who had harmed themselves	There remains considerable uncertainty about which forms of psychosocial and physical treatments for patients who harm themselves are most effective
Ryan (2005)	Studies of any treatment for depression involving children and adolescents with depression	Cognitive behavioural therapy and interpersonal therapy are better than treatment as usual; several antidepressants are more efficacious than placebo; there is a correlation between treatment with SSRIs and a decrease in completed suicide, however comparing all antidepressants as a single group the association is with an increase in suicide

(DBT) showing some promise when used with patients who have borderline personality disorder. This treatment is discussed further in Chapter 7. In the second study, Cowdery *et al.* (1990) reported a case of behaviour therapy to reduce self-harm. A nine-year-old boy substantially decreased the frequency with which he self-mutilated over the course of 50 therapy sessions, using differential reinforcement of other (non-self-harming) behaviour (DRO). He was not reported as having any specific mental health diagnosis.

In summarising the evidence in relation to self-harm and attempted suicide, the Scottish Executive (2008) concluded that there is some evidence that DBT may be of value. However, they note that it is important that future research outcomes relating to the cognitive components of both this therapy and of CBT are distinguished from outcomes attributable solely to the behavioural component. In the same review, there is also some support for the efficacy of ongoing contact.

However, in the context of self-harm, outcomes for this form of intervention are slightly less convincing than is the case for attempted suicide. There is currently no support for the efficacy of GP-based contact and training initiatives or for psychosocial interventions carried out in the context of emergency medical assessment or admission. However, there is some limited evidence for referral to specialist services following acts of self-harm (Scottish Executive 2008).

NICE guidelines

Clinical guidelines are systematic statements about best practice. They are designed to help professionals, health service commissioners and users to make informed decisions about appropriate treatment options for specific conditions. Clinical guidelines published by NICE set standards for the short-term physical and psychological management and secondary prevention of self-harm in primary and secondary care (NICE 2004a).

The guidelines apply to adults and children aged over eight who have self-harmed and their families and carers. The purpose of the guidelines is to improve standards of care, reduce variations in service quality and ensure that children and young people who self-harm receive care, treatment and management that meet their needs. They are intended to build on the knowledge and skills professionals have in recognising and responding appropriately to young people who self-harm. The guidelines are also designed to help develop and maintain high quality support, care and treatment interventions for young people who self-harm and their families or carers.

Focusing on the first 48 hours of care following self-harm, the guidelines evaluate the following areas:

- specific roles of primary and secondary care professionals
- risk assessment and management strategies
- specific psychological and pharmacological interventions
- specific service delivery systems and service led interventions.

The NHS Centre for Reviews and Dissemination (1998) examined effective health care for self-harm and concluded that there is insufficient evidence to recommend a specific clinical intervention. However, several treatments have produced positive outcomes and these are discussed in detail in Chapter 7.

Summary

Although no form of treatment has been found to be effective in stopping or significantly reducing self-harm by children and young people, some interventions appear to address other factors associated with self-harm in this population, such as depression and emotional control (Social Care Institute for Excellence 2005).

Considerable uncertainty exists about which forms of psychosocial and physical treatment are the most effective. It is unlikely that one approach could fit all young people who self-harm. Approaches should be individualised rather than generalised, and packages of care should be based on young people's views and experiences. Some of the more promising treatments for suicidal and self-harming young people will be explored later in the book.

4 What do young people tell us about self-harm?

Key points:

- There is an extensive body of research focusing on the views and opinions of young people who self-harm. It is important that professionals and other adults take full account of this when planning, delivering or evaluating self-harm interventions and services.
- Young people often say that using physical pain is a way of distracting themselves from distressing thoughts and feelings. Indeed, many report that physical pain caused by cutting or burning is easier to deal with than emotional pain.
- The caring professions in particular can be extremely paternalistic and it is not unusual for professionals to want to rescue the young person from their distress and make them better. To do this, professionals may feel they have to stop a young person self-harming. This can be a problem if a young person does not want to stop and can actually make the problem worse.
- According to young people, positive attitudes, being listened to and given time, being treated in a safe environment and being involved in treatment decisions are all important. Rather than professional friends, young people want staff to be friendly professionals.
- Young people often report that support groups are helpful. Self-help groups and peer support programmes have been proposed as potentially effective in providing help to people who self-harm.
- Many young people who self-harm are very creative and use poetry or artwork as a type of replacement skill when their emotions are running high. For some, it helps refocus them and distracts them from intense feelings. For others though, it can trigger self-harming episodes.

Introduction

Despite popular belief, professionals and other adults do not always know what is best for a young person who self-harms. This chapter focuses exclusively on the experiences and views of young people about self-harm. What parents and carers tell us has been kept separate and is discussed later in the book. This chapter is split into three sections. The first describes young people's views about self-harm; the second explores their views about professionals; and the third discusses young people's views about treatments they receive for self-harm.

This chapter places less emphasis on messages from evidence-based practice, which was discussed in Chapter 3. Instead, it focuses more on what we refer to as practice-based evidence – testimonies from suicidal and self-harming young people themselves.

What do young people tell us?

There is a vast literature exploring service user views about self-harm. Although much of this has focused on adults, there have also been numerous investigations and studies involving young people (Arnold 1995; Garcia *et al.* 2007; YoungMinds 2008).

I Feel like I'm Invisible was a report of an 18-month inquiry jointly conducted by the Mental Health Foundation and the Camelot Foundation (Dow 2004). It connects evidence and research about self-harm with policy and good practice recommendations. The report highlights the need for professionals to understand why young people self-harm and what the triggers for this are.

Who's Hurting Who? looked at the views of young people aged between 15 and 25 about self-harm services (Spandler 1996). A key theme that young people reported was the need for control, both of the self-harm and of the meaning this had for them. Young people explained that when control was taken away from them, this often felt like abuse. This had the paradoxical effect of the young person harming themselves more. The report also drew attention to the apparent inability of helping services to accept that for some young people, self-harm is a way of life.

The Opal Project is run by young people, for young people, and is made up of young people who self-harm and their friends. They provide a range of resources for young people, including the *Spectrum Journal* – a catalogue of notes, drawings, poetry and photographs by young people who self-harm. This is in addition to an information pack for parents and professionals, and a range of leaflets and posters that give positive messages about self-harm. *The Opal Project* is also able to provide talks about self-harm and the work of the project. This is for youth groups, organisations working with young people, schools and mental health services.

Researchers in the CASE study asked young people about many things, including bullying and abuse, drug and alcohol use. Relationships with friends and circumstances within their families were also explored. Any significant life event was found to increase the risk of self-harm and, perhaps unsurprisingly, multiple or interrelated events increased their risk further still (Madge *et al.* 2008).

Truth Hurts – *The National Self-harm Inquiry*

One of the most important studies of young people's views about self-harm, *Truth Hurts*, was undertaken by the Mental Health Foundation and Camelot Foundation in 2006. This brought together the available evidence from a range of sources about young people aged between 11 and 25. The Inquiry panel reviewed published literature and heard evidence from more than 35 organisations and individuals concerned with young people and self-harm. Among other things, the report urged professionals and other adults who work with young people to hear the voices of young people (Mental Health Foundation and Camelot Foundation 2006).

Another key source of information is *Understanding Self-harm,* the report of a web-based questionnaire by SANE which explored the views of nearly 1,000 people and respondents were aged between 12 and 60 (SANE 2008). Many of the key insights and messages for professionals contained in *Truth Hurts* and *Understanding Self-harm* and other key reports are included in this chapter. These are illustrated in speech bubbles, as well as several messages from young people which have informed the practice and knowledge of the authors.

Young people's views about self-harm

This chapter is focused on the views of the young people who responded to the National Inquiry and draws on some of their personal testimonies which are referenced throughout the report. Other relevant reports and sources of information are discussed with a specific emphasis on young people's views. The concluding paragraphs include the personal material and stories of young people who attended an outpatient programme in a Tier 4 service in the north-west of England.

The National Inquiry focused on the journey of the young person from their first episode of self-harm, their experiences of services and ultimately recovery for some of the young people. There are many interpretations of why young people self-harm from the clinical and research literature but the strength of the Inquiry was how it captured descriptions from the young people themselves.

> Self-harm used to be a way to get rid of feelings inside of me, to get out all the hurt, anger and pain that I was feeling. The rush is gone; the sense of feeling better was always so short-lived, so short that I was doing it many times. I've been through times when I haven't been able to get up in the morning and function during the day without self-harm, but not now. Now the longer I can manage without it, the better. I'm trying to get my life 'normal'.

Here are some of those personal testimonies about self-harming. Several statements were made by young people who did not give evidence to the National Inquiry. The statements from young people illustrate an important distinction. They imply that rather than an attempt to take one's life, self-harm is often a way of taking control of and surviving the stresses of life.

> It seems crazy but although my friends and family felt I was out of control I felt I was in control. Like I had found it again through self-harming.

> Just like scar tissue that you might have now, it doesn't tan in the sun because it's dead. If you hurt inside for whatever reason, your insides will die and you don't feel anything but your brain still works, you are still physically alive and the only way to bring those feelings back is to physically feel something.

These extracts suggest that self-harm brings around a sense of relief from tension and enables a balancing of emotions. Smith *et al.* (1998) express how neurochemicals play an important role in self-harm. Following a release of endogenous opioids, commonly known as endorphins, people who self-harm often experience a sense of relief. These chemicals are released by the pituitary gland and hypothalamus when the body is injured in any way and they dampen down sensitivity to pain that will help the individual survive. Furthermore, people can become addicted to the release of these opioids and thus a greater level of self-harm may have to be inflicted to achieve the same effect. This biological perspective also implies that the endorphin release can provide an escape from what is felt to be unbearable pain.

> I feel a warm sense of relief as though all the bad things about me were flowing out of me and made me feel alive, real.

> Sometimes when I felt numb and empty, scratching myself helped me to feel emotions again. Brought me back to life in a way.

Serotonin is a neurotransmitter which is also implicated in self-harm. It is released when a person is subjected to high levels of stress. Some have suggested that being exposed to stress produces lower levels of serotonin over time. Low levels of serotonin can be linked to impulsive risk-taking behaviour and, since people who self-harm are often impulsive, it may be harder for those who already self-harm to resist the urge to do it again (Nav *et al.* 2005; Madge *et al.* 2008).

> I don't deal with daily stress well, so when extra events occur, however big or small, my tension levels rise resulting in my needing to 'release'. Self-harm has proven to be most successful in dealing with this.

Self-harm also helps some young people regulate distressing 'self states', such as dissociation. This involves a disruption in what are usually integrated functions of consciousness, memory, identity, or perception of the environment, which may be sudden or gradual, transient or chronic (American Psychiatric Association 1994). It has been suggested that some young people harm themselves in order to feel 'real', and that a form of dissociation ensues following the act which enables the young person to connect back to the here and now (Low *et al.* 2000; Farber 2008; Bracken *et al.* 2008).

> At the same time as feeling numb I felt extreme pain, so I cut and it got rid of the feeling. Cutting in small amounts doesn't usually help me to relieve pain. It used to but I've done it for so long I need to cut a lot to help it now.

> If I had never cut myself I probably still wouldn't be around today.

Much has been written about the way self-harm enables people to use physical pain as a way to distract oneself from distressing thoughts and feelings. Indeed, many young people feel that physical pain caused by cutting or burning is easier to deal with than emotional pain (Mental Health Foundation and Camelot Foundation 2006). It can also be a means of punishing oneself for perceived misdemeanours.

> My emotions vary rapidly and can be very intense. In an emotionally charged situation, I will either, during or shortly after, harm myself. I'm not good at dealing with emotions or communicating mine to others.

Another, more recent, report conduced by SANE (2008) provided some qualitative evidence about the reasons young people self-harm. Table 4.1 illustrates some of the reasons young people give for their first and subsequent acts of self-harm.

Table 4.1 Motivation for self-harm (from SANE 2008)

By accident	'It was an accident. I dropped something on my hand and it was like a light coming on. I felt something at last. It felt really refreshing like I had learned something new and important.'
During a suicide attempt	'I was intending to commit suicide but found relief from just one cut.'
In the context of self-harm aimed at eliciting a response from others	'The first time I self-injured was a different situation to those which followed. I self-injured in order to avoid a violent punishment.'
When the primary motivation for harm was self-punishment or expression of self-loathing	'First I did it to punish myself for not doing well in exams, then I did it because I wanted everything to stop.'

Many participants in the SANE (2008) research had long histories of self-harm and some had begun self-harming at the age of four. Whilst some people report using self-harm compulsively, or to connect with their feelings, this was not the case for them. Rather, respondents had experienced a number of distressing experiences and used self-harm to bring about a sense of relief from the accumulation. A surprising number of people did not know why they self-harmed or felt that they had self-harmed without reason. Others described a type of 'hidden self'.

> When others find me attractive or pretty or socially appealing I harm a lot more because I know that they are wrong and I am right and that I have a dark rotten core.

Another response describes this notion further:

> I have to behave as if my feelings, beliefs and thoughts are different from what they actually are.

Young people hide their behaviour for various reasons. Some fear being a burden, whilst others are concerned about hurting or frightening their friends and family. Young people gave a range of explanations to SANE about why their hid their self-harm from others. These included feeling judged or condemned, and not wanting to explain or answer questions. Failing expectations was a specific issue and referred primarily to relapse of their self-harm. The most common motivation reported to SANE was to relieve mental pain with over half of all respondents citing this as their primary reason.

> Sometimes my emotional pain is so strong that I don't feel I can take it and that it's going to destroy me. I just know I need to stop it. Cutting my arms seems to help me do that.

As part of their research, SANE launched a website questionnaire charting the journey from the first to final acts of self-harm by young people who had recovered. The age range included older people, however, the majority of respondents were below 25 years. For most, their self-harm had taken place during early or late adolescence. The research team asked open-ended questions and interpreted what the participants said. Some of the extracts are shown below:

> First I did it to punish myself for not doing well in exams then I did it because I wanted everything to stop.

> The first time I self-injured was a different situation to those which followed. I self-injured to avoid a punishment.

> I had heard about people doing this when they were depressed and wanted to see how it would make me feel.

> When I feel empty it's like there is nothing inside me. I'd do anything to fill that gaping hole. I used to stuff myself with food but it was never enough but when I cut it just goes.

Learning from others

Without doubt, issues of contagion are present where groups of young people live together. This issue was discussed in the first two chapters. Contagion frequently affects self-harm when the groups of children and young people typically have backgrounds of trauma, abuse and neglect. This is partly why there is an increased prevalence of self-harm in children's homes, mental health inpatient settings and prisons. Some argue that this problem is made worse due to scarce resources and competing demands for staff support. The young person who does not self-harm may come to observe that there are more benefits for their peers who self-harm in terms of individual staff support time. The effects of peer group relationships on self-harming behaviour and on reaching resolution is an area which requires further research and attention.

> The first time I self-harmed was in a mental hospital so everyone else around me was doing it. I kind of picked up the habit off them.

Just over a quarter of participants with a history of self-harm stated they had stopped. Commonly, people reported that they stopped self-harming not because they wanted to, but rather as a result of social pressure.

> I still miss it and would continue if the scars were not so hard to hide and long in fading.

Some young people told researchers that they had stopped self-harming to accommodate changes in their role. Becoming a parent, an employee, wife or husband led some to stop. Others said they didn't want to go on upsetting people such as their parents.

> My parents found out and made me feel bad about it. I'm glad I don't do it any more but only because I don't want to upset anyone.

Stopping for some was linked to the maturational process. They reported growing in confidence, increased stability and more control over their lives. One account from a young person was that of being given permission, so to speak.

> After I'd been in hospital, I went to the college nurse and told her I had been self-harming. She told me that there was nothing wrong with doing it and that I should continue if I wanted to and booked me into see a counsellor. By telling me that I could do it, it took the guilt out of the cycle and I slowly began to stop. I finally realised that what I was doing wasn't 'bad' or wrong it was just my way of coping.

This type of permissiveness may be an important element in encouraging young people to manage their self-harm. They sometimes experience a sense of self-loathing after an episode, and are left with similar emotions precipitating the act. Therefore, for some it may be a way of intervening positively in the vicious circle that young people often find themselves in. Conversely, some will stop because they feel guilt before and after self-harming.

Young people's views about professionals

Various professionals in both statutory and voluntary sector services are involved in helping young people who self-harm. Whilst many young people have positive experiences of being cared for by staff, others have a negative experience. *Truth Hurts* painted a bleak picture at times. Young people told the Inquiry that the experience of asking for help often made their situation worse. Many of them were met with ridicule or hostility from the professionals they had turned to (Mental Health Foundation and Camelot Foundation 2006). In a qualitative study of self-harm by Smith (2002), patients reported that adults often did not understand their behaviour or feelings. They reported that staff treated them like naughty children and made those who return to hospital following further acts of self-harm feel like failures.

> After I cut myself I feel good, like I've punished them, secretly. I can be talking to them and I can feel my arm and it's like 'stuff you', like I've got one over on them.

Children and young people often have difficulty explaining their feelings and problems to others. They may not have the vocabulary to describe what is happening to them to the extent that many do not even ask for help. Mental health difficulties often go unrecognised or get passed off as teenage angst. Views expressed by adults that they will 'grow out of it' can erect barriers to communication and prevent access to professional help. Adults may, for example, assume that the child or young person is simply passing through a stage. Indeed they are, but for some they require help in navigating this stage. Minimising their distress can result in the young person becoming isolated.

> She told me I should stop being selfish and think of my parents. She asked me what I would think if they died.

Adults may be alarmed by a teenager who talks about suicide and may use statements such as 'you shouldn't talk like that' or 'don't be silly you have your whole life in front of you'. Whilst well intended, such comments are often perceived by young people as unhelpful. The caring professions in particular can be extremely paternalistic and it is not unusual for staff to want to rescue the young person from their distress and make them better. To do this, professionals may feel they have to extinguish a young person's self-harming behaviour.

This can be a problem if a young person does not want to stop. Indeed, some youngsters have said they do not want to stop self-harming as it performs an important and worthwhile function for them and does not harm anyone else. The natural instinct for people in the caring professions is compromised when the young person rejects help or does not want to reduce their self-harming behaviour. Young people report that having their means of self-harm taken away from them may result in them finding alternative ways of harming themselves, such as not eating.

> I have learned not to tell people when I self-harm because they will only want me to stop. I will only end up burning myself. I need to show on my skin all the hurt inside. I can be talking to you but when I feel my arm it's like my body and I can decide what to do with me.

Being dismissed or disbelieved may also mean that the young person chooses not to verbalise their feelings. Instead, they may attempt to cope alone with what are often extremely frightening emotions. Initial responses by professionals to self-harm disclosures are crucial in engaging the young people in treatment. It is therefore imperative that professionals and other adults are mindful of these potentially counter therapeutic approaches.

The poem below is written by a girl who was admitted to hospital following self-harm. It describes her unhelpful experience of conflict within a staff group.

Conflict, by Laura

I sit here thinking about my miserable life
Knowing that relief would come if you'd give me the knife
There is no chance of a silent tear
The staff don't realise it's all a bluff
And that deep inside I am not very tough
You all pretend that you care
But all you do is sit and stare
I've changed so much in so little time
Look at me now I used to be fine
My life no longer has any meaning
So recognise that I am actually screaming
I don't want you to feel annoyed at me
Because you can't fix what you really can't see

Laura describes the dichotomy involving her need to be cared for and the inability of staff to see beyond her façade. Undoubtedly, it can be difficult for some professionals to avoid withdrawal or avoidance, at least temporarily, when faced with someone who is deliberately inflicting damage on themselves.

However, negativism by staff can foster hopelessness for the young person which is what Laura seems to be portraying in the poem.

One of the key questions asked of young people by the National Inquiry was 'what do you think could be done to help prevent young people from feeling that they want to hurt themselves?' Over a quarter of the respondents said that they wanted someone who would listen to them and give advice and support. The Inquiry highlighted some of the work done by the charity *The Place 2BE* in early intervention. This charity provides a dedicated team to work with young people within the school environment in a room referred to as a 'safe space'. The workers provide training for the school workforce in both identifying and addressing unmet emotional needs.

> The Head didn't want me to mess up the league tables so she told my mum about self-harm and soon everyone in the school knew but no one could give me any real support because my role was to concentrate on getting A* for the school.

It is not new that there is much evidence commenting on the growing unhappiness among young people who are striving to deal with the challenges of our modern day society. Research from the children's charity NSPCC reports that between 2002 and 2003 over 3,000 children and young people called their counsellors about self-harm or suicidal thoughts (NSPCC 2007). A more recent survey by ChildLine shows that figures have tripled in the last five years to an average of nearly 60 a week. Over half of all the calls about self-harm are from children aged between 12 and 15, and 16 times as many girls than boys call for help (NSPCC 2009).

Views of accident and emergency staff

For many young people, their first formal contact following an episode of self-harm is with their local accident and emergency (A&E) department. Much has been written about the important role of A&E professionals and some of this is discussed in Chapter 9. Whilst attendance at hospital following self-harm can be the first stage in accessing help and moving towards recovery, the process can also be fraught with difficulties.

The young person presenting at A&E is likely to be distressed, confused and frightened, and the way in which the staff respond will clearly influence their engagement and experience of health care. Many staff are helpful, understanding and able to support the young person during their distress, but on too many occasions research has shown that this is not the case. The Royal College of Psychiatrists surveyed 509 people of all ages who attended A&E departments following an episode of self-harm. They found that a substantial number of patients had been blamed for wasting time as staff considered that their problems had been 'self-inflicted' (Palmer *et al.* 2007).

> I have not self-harmed in order to annoy staff but rather because something is very, very wrong inside.

According to Fortune *et al.* (2005), the majority of adolescents believe that they can cope on their own, and choose not to engage with professionals. This may be as much about personal choice as the belief that professionals are not competent to help them. In many cases they may be right. Other young people who self-harm talk about wanting to be looked after by caring staff. The following quote is taken from the *Basement Project*, a service for people who have been abused as children and those who self-harm:

> It gave me an excuse to go to the nurse and be bandaged up and taken care of.

This may be one reason the pejorative phrase 'attention-seeking behaviour' has become inextricably linked to self-harm in the minds of many. Young people have stated that in some instances they have self-harmed to communicate to others that they are distressed and that they have wanted to feel cared for and looked after. We have heard that it is part of human nature to seek positive attention from others, and some young people struggle to do this more than others. Responses to young people who self-harm should not be punitive or over parental. Rather, it is important to respond as a friendly professional and not as a professional friend. Maintaining a helpful, optimistic therapeutic alliance and healthy interpersonal boundary is imperative when the young person's life may appear incredibly bleak (Burke *et al.* 2008).

> What they fail to consider is that maybe a young person simply needs someone to talk to, not specifically about self-harm but about the problems and issues they are facing in their daily lives which makes them turn to self-harm as a way of simply surviving.

Some of the personal testimonies described in the National Inquiry and in various other reports, including NICE guidelines on self-harm, describe negative and sometimes hostile reactions from A&E staff. Although this is unacceptable, A&E staff often describe feeling inadequately qualified to support young people who self-harm. It is therefore crucial that better training, supervision and support for this key part of the children's workforce is available. The following are examples of some young people's experiences of feeling like time wasters.

> The doctor didn't speak English but he was still able to convey his disgust with me. I could see it in his face and he certainly didn't want to be bothered with me.

> I was covered in blood and the admitting staff let me sit in the crowded waiting area. They didn't even give me eye contact. Another patient gave me some tissues and spoke to me softly.

> As if I didn't feel crap enough, the student nurse who wasn't much older then me cleaned my wounds without even speaking to me. She made me feel like a piece of dirt from under her finger nails.

Young people's views of services

As well as their experiences of individual professionals, various consultation exercises have been undertaken to elicit young people's views about the services they receive. A project for young people aged between 13 and 25 in Leeds sought to understand the factors that make services for self-harm effective (Neill 2003). Confidentiality, having choice and being respected were identified as important factors.

> My nurse would spend loads of time teaching me alternative strategies when I felt the urge to self-harm. I had drawn up a safety plan with her which I carried in my bag. I had a list of other things to do and she was so kind and without her I don't know if I would get through that horrible time in my life.

Young people's views about self-management

We have heard that many young people who self-harm do not want professional help and prefer to cope alone or within friendship circles. Much has been written about self-management and the importance of the young person being able to distract themselves from self-harming. Some of these techniques which are reported by young people to be helpful are highlighted at the end of this chapter. One form of self-management which a lot of young people rate highly is the technique of postponing the urge to self-harm in the knowledge that the feelings will more than likely pass. One young person who spoke to the National Inquiry described this eloquently:

> I tried so many things, from holding ice cubes, elastic band flicking on the wrist, writing down my thoughts, hitting a pillow, listening to music, writing down pros and cons, but the most helpful to my recovery was the five minute rule where if you feel like you want to self-harm you wait for five minutes before you do, then see if you can go another five minutes and so on until eventually the urge is over.

Some young people describe managing their self-harm by developing different coping skills. An initial stage of effective self-management appears to involve understanding why one self-harms. In a sense, having the knowledge is power. Importantly and positively, a lot of young people believe their recovery is enhanced by learning self-management skills.

For some young people who self-harm, insight into the reasons why they do so is liberating and an essential part of coping, whereas others find the development of coping strategies essential during their recovery. The Mental Health Foundation and Camelot Foundation produced a questionnaire asking young people about treatments that had not been helpful. A substantial number of young people who were unable to disclose their self-harming behaviour gave the following reasons:

> They would think I was crazy like some screwball kid who was just a nuisance and playing some sicko games.

> I expect they would give me sympathy, which would make the feelings worse.

> They could be supportive but not know what to do and that would make things worse. Then everybody else would find out.

Support from family and friends

During adolescence, peer group relationships often become more intense and have a strong influence on the development of interests, beliefs and behaviour. Whilst young people may be less inclined to talk to their parents or carers, they may share their worries or concerns with friends. Research has shown that those who disclose their self-harm to friends are younger than those who share these with their family (SANE 2008). This was supported by young people who gave evidence to the National Inquiry. They were three times more likely to suggest talking to friends or family than professionals.

Previous studies have consistently shown that girls and young women are more likely to do this than boys and young men (Adams *et al.* 1995; Fivush *et al.* 2004; Madge *et al.* 2008).

Friends and peers have an important role to play in helping to identify and support those who are vulnerable. Studies have examined the social relationships of young people who have taken an overdose, and a somewhat mixed picture emerges. Half say that they have no 'close' or 'best' friend, and this is more likely in boys (Kerfoot 1988). Since it is often best friends that young people confide in, this is a clearly a concern at a number of levels.

> They would support me, as most of my friends have mental problems I take their problems and it helps me cope, so they can know mine.

Listening and supporting are important friendship qualities, but if the problems cannot be influenced or resolved within friendship circles, they may continue or worsen. Here, the support of parents, carers or professionals may be warranted. Within peer group relationships this often raises issues of loyalty and trust. Friends find themselves in a dilemma about 'telling' or sharing information in an attempt to enlist support for their friend. The absence of a supportive peer group may compound difficulties which can build up over time. In such circumstances, young people may feel as if problems have become insurmountable. A crisis may then ensue and self-harm may become an option.

The nature of adolescence is often characterised by a mistrust of adults and the young person's friend can often be more informed about the likely precipitating factors, extent of self-harm and possibly some of the maintaining factors. A very young self-harming girl expressed her thoughts about her friend who also self-harms:

> She is the only one who understands. She doesn't judge or blow her top. She accepts me for who I am and without her in my life I would not be able to stop.

Conversely, the friends of young people who self-harm may be misguided and get out of their depth in either keeping the secret or feeling responsible for the friend's inability to stop. These types of dialogue take place interpersonally and across the many internet sites, and require careful management for both parties.

> Maria needed help but she made me promise I wouldn't tell her parents. She wasn't ill or anything it was just her mood, I didn't think she would actually cut herself. I wished I hadn't made the promise now.

Vulnerable young people have a tendency to take on other's troubles and it is unlikely that they are able to differentiate between what is psychological distress and what is simply part of adolescence. The situation may be further complicated if the young person she tells is self-harming themselves. This is a concerning yet common dialogue between self-harmers. However, it is also worrying as young people often feel a certain loyalty and may keep suicidal plans about others to themselves. When young people engage quite intensely with fellow self-harmers the relationship is a salient factor to be addressed for both.

It is natural that young people will seek out like-minded peers. Even if adults dissuade them from particular relationships, the young person may rebel against the advice. The experience of clinicians is that young people who self-harm will find each other, whether permitted to or not, and the relationship is highly likely to continue, whether covertly or overtly.

One of the main avenues young people communicate about self-harm is though Facebook and MSN chat rooms. They may feel very intensely and intimately involved with fellow self-harmers, and inevitably share experiences both positive and negative. However, left unchecked, these relationships may sometimes have a mutually negative effect. For this reason, some have argued that grouping young people who self-harm together in a more controlled way may be effective (Wood *et al.* 2001).

Alienation

The influence of friends and family is not always perceived by young people as helpful. An American study by Young and Gunderson (1995) looked at the families of 55 young people aged 14 to 18 who had been admitted to an inpatient adolescent unit. Two-thirds of the cohort was suicidal and all had shown what the researchers called 'self-destructive' behaviour. The study made comparisons between the views of young people and those of their parents. It was reported that those who were more suicidal tended to see themselves as more alienated from their parents, more socially isolated and as having poorer overall functioning than others. Their parents did not concur, which to some extent supported the young people's perception that they were alienated.

What is the role of support groups?

Young people often report that support groups are helpful. Self-help groups and peer support programmes have been proposed as potentially effective in providing help to people who self-harm (Social Care Institute for Excellence 2005). The National Self-harm Network (NSHN) provides support and advice to people who self-harm, as well as their friends and family. Harmless is a user-led organisation that provides a range of services about self-harm, including support, information, training and consultancy to people who self-harm, their friends and families and professionals.

The pros and cons of support groups have been debated for some time, and there are certainly personal testimonies to the attractiveness of groups for young people. This is particularly the helpfulness of contact with peers who have had similar experiences. Being part of a group is an adolescent phenomenon, and as youngsters who self-harm can often feel excluded from their peers, the group can provide them with an inclusive experience. Careful orchestration by the facilitators can ensure that the group is a positive, corrective experience and it has proven clinical utility (Wood *et al.* 2001). However, many professionals have reservations about this modality and are concerned that talking about self-harm to other people who self-harm may encourage people to continue, and to self-harm in new ways (Clarke 2003).

Self-harm management strategies that young people find helpful

Since for many young people self-harm is a private activity, it is crucially important that they can develop strategies to cope alone. The remainder of this chapter focuses on material provided by a group of young people aged 11–18 who repeatedly self-harm. This is used to illustrate how young people develop self-management strategies to live with, and sometimes combat, self-harm. Approximately three-quarters of the young people who contributed the material regularly overdosed or cut themselves, and a minority used other methods, such as hanging, strangulation and burning. All the young people attended a group treatment programme called Developmental Group Psychotherapy (DGP), which was described in Chapter 3.

The young people formed an extremely heterogeneous group. Some chose current material, such as songs, to describe their experience, and several provided artwork, which included some graphic drawings of wounds and blood. Although many people find such artwork disturbing, graphic drawings or artwork are a common medium among people who self-harm.

Some young people prefer to write down their feelings rather than act them out. This may help distance themselves from the immediacy of the experience. Others may prefer vigorous physical activity to distract themselves from self-harm. The following are some of the titles of the young people's work.

- 'All the platitudes about loss getting better with time – it doesn't actually'
- 'It's not a bitter rivalry'
- 'I looked in the mirror and hated myself'
- 'Up close and personal'
- 'Inside story'
- 'Angels and Airwaves'

Self-harm and poetry

Many young people who self-harm are very creative and use poetry or art-work as a type of replacement skill when their emotions are running high. For some, it helps refocus them and distracts them from intense feelings. For others, it can trigger self-harming episodes. An open discourse about the communication may be helpful given that young people use creativity and art for different reasons.

Angels and Airwaves, by Kirsty

She was a wingless angel
She was a beauty hidden behind sorrow
Nothing made sense in her upside down world
No one held out a hand for her to hold it seems she just fell forever
Her wings were taken right from her back
She was a wingless angel
Perhaps he did love her
Suppose they were meant to be
So why did he love her and let her fall
Where did he go when she needed him most?
This world was so unfaithful to her
She was but an angel who lost her wings
She was a most precious stone
Hidden deep and fair in the darkest of caves
She wanted only to find her way
To be a someone
Why could they not help her?
She just needed help in finding her wings

Kirsty's poem communicates her isolation and desire to be rescued. Referring to herself as a 'wingless angel' perhaps depicts the inertia of entrapment that surrounds her. The words appear to oscillate between the intolerable feelings of hopelessness without her wings, and Kirsty's desire for someone to provide for her or help her find her wings.

Penny is 15 years of age and began self-harming when she was eight. She has a history of abuse and has taken very serious overdoses over the past year. She struggles to communicate her inner turmoil and uses prose, art and poetry to compensate for her lack of verbal communication. Her poem on page 97 expresses her wish to be saved from drifting too far. She expresses ambivalence about her plight and whether she can be saved in time.

Nancy is 17 years of age and has a long term history of self-harming behaviour and she describes how it started and about the many reinforcing factors alluding to the addictive quality of the behaviour. Nancy's poem ends up acknowledging that the course is as yet undecided.

Think, by Nancy

I feel sad and lonely,
I need a way to let it all out,
My friend used to cut herself,
She said she felt better,
She's stopped now though,
Maybe it will help me,
I start to cry,
I feel so depressed,
I can hear something inside my head saying
'Do it, do it'
Whispering,
Egging me on,
I wipe my tears away,
They are a sign of weakness,
I will show no one my weakness,
I decide I shall try it
I go to my kitchen,
As dimly lighted as it may be,
I draw closer to the draw,
I open it,
Out comes a collection of cutlery,
My hand reaches for the first sharpest knife I see,
I pick it up,
The metal is cold and smooth,
The blade is sharp,
This knife is small,
So this will do nicely,
I go back into my room,
And press the ice-cold blade against my warm skin,
I press down and drag,
A searing pain comes from dragging the blade,
The pain numbs my mind, and I can feel again,
And think clearly,
I do it agin and again,
And when I finally stop,
I have many gashes on my wrist,
I look and think,
I do actually feel better,
But I won't do it again, I mustn't
Although I feel better I will always have these to remind me of my pain,
But as time heals them,
It will heal a peace inside of me,
And I will be able to move on,

Finally,
But even though I said never again,
Every night I still rip open my flesh,
Every time there was more,
And were deeper,
So before you think
'Let me do it just once'
Don't as even though it helps,
It's very hard to stop,
You may end up doing it for a majority of your life,
You honestly never know.

Nearly noticed, by Penny

She is lonely
Even though you can't tell
She is reaching out
For what, she doesn't know
She will sit in silence
Hoping for someone to stumble across her and all her emptiness
But they only hope that they do it in time
Otherwise she will have drifted too far
And may have to let go of whatever grasps of the world she has
As she will slowly fade out of the lives of everyone
She repeats to herself 'Nearly noticed'

Self-harm and music

Young people often prefer to use the medium of art and music as a way of expressing feelings that they find difficult to verbalise. In particular, song lyrics are frequently associated with individual meaning. Two songs by the American rock group Linkin Park, 'Breaking the habit' and 'Somewhere I belong' are examples, chosen by young people, they contain lyrics which depict very eloquently the struggle of beating self-harm and the internal battle that often ensues between life and death.

Security management plans

As stated earlier, a central tenet in the treatment of self-harm involves self-management. Many young people value their individualised security plan, which can be revised as techniques or strategies become less potent.

As part of formulating the plan, young people select coping strategies which may include alternatives to self-harm, and often focus on harm minimisation, which is a risk management approach discussed in Chapter 7. Although currently there is no robust evidence to confirm the positive effects of individual security planning, it ensures that the young person is an active participant in their own recovery. A list of things young people reported they found to be helpful as a distraction from the urge to self-harm is shown below.

- Stay in a public place
- Be with safe and supportive people
- Call a friend
- Write in a journal
- Watch a funny movie
- Make a no harm contract with your therapist
- Go for a drive
- Do relaxation exercises
- Do deep breathing
- Listen to music
- Read a good book
- Go for a walk
- Clean
- Take a bubble bath
- Go shopping
- Wear a rubber band around your wrist and when the urge to harm is strong, snap it lightly
- Hold ice in your hand
- Use a washable red pen and make marks where you want to hurt yourself
- Get rid of anything you could hurt yourself with

Dealing with strong emotions

Young people also identify ways in which they attempt to cope with strong emotions, such as anger and sadness, or feelings of emptiness and guilt. These, of course, are also regarded by many young people as alternatives to self-harm in themselves. The logic behind many of these strategies is that when young people feel emotionally aroused they often have a lot of energy. The alternatives provide ways to release that energy without causing harm.

Recognising the emotions that precipitate self-harming urges often means that coping skills are more effective. Like the strategies to replace destructive self-harm with less harmful coping mechanisms, the ways in which young people attempt to manage strong emotions will vary. Indeed, some strategies may make a young person feel worse, and promoting them as helpful may actually increase their destructive self-harming behaviour.

The following extract gives some examples of techniques that young people use to deal with strong feelings and urges. These were cited in The National Inquiry and have been endorsed in other research reports and in service user testimonies. The goals of these techniques are to help moderate impulsive behaviour and regulate emotions. Of course the list is not exhaustive, and what is helpful for one young person may not be an acceptable alternative to self-harm for another.

Managing strong feelings

Anger

- Squeeze ice
- Do something that will give you a sharp sensation, like biting a lemon
- Exercise
- Take a walk
- Crumple pieces of paper; rip them up
- Take a cold shower
- Imagine getting even with the person who is making you angry or upset
- Listen to angry music; sing along, dance
- Scream loudly
- Snap a rubber band against your wrist
- Cry – this releases emotions as well as making you feel drained and tired and if you sleep, things will usually seem better when you wake up
- Beat up something that isn't alive, like a pillow
- Play a musical instrument, or bang pots and pans
- Cut up cardboard or an old piece of clothing or fabric
- Flatten aluminium cans for recycling
- Pick up a stick and hit a tree

Sadness

- Take a bath, put bubbles in it
- Read a book that you like; read a children's book – they always have happy endings
- Buy yourself a present
- Watch a funny movie
- Watch cartoons
- Go out somewhere with a friend
- Write, draw, play a musical instrument – express yourself creatively
- Hug a toy animal
- Hug a loved one
- Hug yourself

- Do something that you loved to do when you were younger
- Read jokes or funny stories – you can find lots of those online
- Talk with a friend – you don't have to talk about self-harm, talk about something cheerful
- Think about things that make you happy and make a list
- Curl up under your duvet
- Listen to cheerful or calming music
- Play with a pet or sibling

Emptiness

- Do something that will give you a sharp sensation, like biting a lemon or squeezing ice
- Focus on one thing. Try to describe it like you would to a blind person
- Put a finger or a hand into frozen food like ice cream
- Put your hands under cold water; take a cold shower
- Focus on your breath, on how your chest and stomach move when you breathe in and out. If you were not real you would not be breathing
- Eat something mindfully. Pay attention to how it tastes and the sensations that it creates in your mouth. Try to describe it to someone who has no sense of taste
- List as many different uses as you can for a random object. Give yourself a number to reach – like 20, 40 or 50. Try to surpass that number. Don't stop after two or three uses
- Interact with other people

Feeling guilty or like a bad person

- List as many good things about yourself as you can. Give yourself a number to reach – like 20, 40 or 50. Try to surpass that number. Don't stop after a few good things
- Read something good that someone has written about you like a letter, a recommendation or an evaluation
- Talk with someone who cares about you
- Do something nice for someone else
- Remember times when you did something good
- What are you feeling guilty about? Can you change it somehow? Try talking with the person you feel guilty towards. Maybe they don't feel as bad as you think they do
- If you want to hurt yourself to punish yourself, punish yourself by not allowing yourself to self-injure instead

Managing addiction

- Draw or write on yourself with a red pen or marker
- Paint yourself with red paint
- Squeeze ice
- Snap a rubber band against your wrist
- Cry
- Exercise
- Buy a cheap tattoo, the kind that comes off after a few days and put it on yourself
- Look at your old scars. This may trigger you more, so be careful. It may also make the urge go away because you are seeing and experiencing scars even though they are old
- The point here is to create feelings and sensations similar to those you experience while hurting yourself. Some of these things create visual images like those you may want to see like scars or blood. Others release endorphins which is what happens when you hurt yourself and what gives you the feeling of euphoria

Waiting

- Play the 15 minute game. Tell yourself 'I will not hurt myself for 15 minutes'
- Pick a favourite singer or band and tell yourself that you will not hurt yourself whilst listening to them
- Pick a day of the week and don't hurt yourself on that day. Eventually add a second day, and then a third, and so on
- Buy a calendar and give yourself a sticker for every day that you don't hurt yourself
- Pick a place to be your safe place, a place you won't cut, like the kitchen, your room etc. Go there when you have an urge
- The idea is to wait before hurting yourself … the urge may go away or be easier to deal with later

Experts by experience

The final words in this chapter are from an 18-year-old girl who has a long-term history of self-harm and eating disordered behaviour who attended a specialist self-harm outpatient service. She has stopped self-harming and is undergoing plastic surgery to reduce her scarring. She now provides consultation and direct support to parents and professionals. Her personal story elucidates the nature of and some motives for her self-injury. In the following extract, Fay pays particular attention to distinguishing her self-harm from suicide, and throughout her story makes reference to the overwhelming depressive thoughts that were, and at times still are, part of her life.

Fay's testimony

There will be a consummate list somewhere of every traditional, origi-nal and creative method to damage yourself. Even smoking, getting wrecked and jacking up once in a while will be up there. This said, the majority of people will harm themselves in some way at some time in their life, with or without intent – maybe without even realising. Those who deliberately hurt themselves have, in essence, just stepped up the deleterious behaviour and made, whatever method intentionally harm-ful to themselves – just like binge drinking, binge eating and smoking.

Self-harm is harmful pain rather than harmful pleasure. I can't speak for everyone obviously but to cut, burn or bruise yourself, at least for me, isn't and wasn't for pleasure. There tends to be a far more negative motive under the plasters. The act of self-injury can provide numerous voices for innumerable emotions and feelings. It holds many different meanings, feelings and functions for that self.

As I saw it, there was no other way to describe or understand the unfath-omable depths of what I was feeling. It was alien to me, it hurt desperately and without anything tangible to tackle I put my mind to my skin instead, in a futile effort to express what I couldn't say. This was making my body become my voice. I didn't bother or hurt anyone else. I was fixing it.

Initially, it was a long lasting quick fix that would get me through the night or day. I think I was about 12 when I took to my arm with a pair of nail scissors. The cuts were superficial. A smattering of blood and a little stinging and it was done. A feeling of intense relief flushed through me. The preced-ing months had been calorie-counted and calculated. I'd starved to gain some control over a life that I thought was falling apart right under my feet.

In the beginning, the starvation was never about weight loss, it was about self-destruction and the juxtaposed self-preservation as I recklessly grabbed at anything that could help. I'd lost myself somewhere along the way. This blanket of depression had settled itself heavily on my shoulders without warning, or apparent trigger, and little Miss A* student didn't have a clever enough answer. She didn't know how to fix it.

After a while, its enchanting efficiency makes it a wholly plausible act to indulge in. As you position your sleeve out of the blood stream, the feelings of guilt and shame dissipate quickly. Self-harm is bitter-sweet. Perversely, like a Swiss army knife, it's multi-purpose. At times I cut to ground myself or in an effort to come back from whatever disso-ciative state I was lingering in. Sometimes it was about survival – other times about purging my sins. Sometimes it was purely a release, like the exhalation of breath, it became natural.

I remember past conversations with my GP when he was patching up my latest curative handiwork. In the end, he thought, in part, that

I'd become addicted. Whether to the actual act, the rush, the result, or what, I do not know, but I've since read about the endorphin argument.

I guess in the end, self-harm even becomes a reasonable response. If you forget what caused the bleeding, burns or broken bones for a moment, it becomes acceptable. A simple cut can be fixed with a plaster. It can be nursed, tended and cared for. This is all technically within the bounds of sane human understanding. If you cut yourself on the bread knife innocently when cooking, your mum will whip out her first aid kit and kiss it better, but if you cut yourself intentionally on that bread knife, there's confusion around whether it's the first aid kit or the psychiatrist you need.

Something to point out about self-harm is that it is not a suicide attempt. In some ways, it's an attempt to stop suicide, or at least delay it. There are so many rumours and misconceptions surrounding this taboo subject. To turn on yourself, you seemingly need to be mad, dangerous, attention seeking, unfeeling and/or manipulative. I'm none of these things, but neither am I the oddball exception.

My self-harm continued for five years. I stopped just after my 17th birthday. In time, the rush had worn off. This admittedly crude tool had ceased to work, and again, I was alone. Since then, my depressions have worsened. Everything's worsened. Proof perhaps that painting over the cracks doesn't repair the damage. Today, I'm left with bad hypertrophic scarring that, I'm told, will need plastic surgery and even then I'll still be scarred.

That first, frenzied fix became my life for half a decade. Even now I've given up my razors, I'm still suffering the after-effects and am still considered one of those mad, dangerous, attention seeking, unfeeling manipulative folk that no one seems able to understand.

Summary

It is not easy to represent the views of children and young people because there is no typical person who self-harms. Different people harm themselves for different reasons and at different times. Some people who self-harm say it is difficult, if not impossible, for people without personal experience to fully understand the issue. However, they believe it is important to listen, to try to understand and, most importantly, not to make assumptions or judge people.

Young people tell us that their friends are important and that they often find it easier to talk to them about self-harm than professionals or parents. In terms of what works for young people who self-harm, they say that continuity and the offer of longer-term interventions are important. They also want staff involved to be non-judgemental, accepting and genuinely interested in them.

The first part of any dialogue begins with the intital stages of assessment. The next chapter explores the assessment of young people's psychosocial needs.

5   Making sense of self-harm

The process of assessment

Key points:

- All professionals are expected to make an assessment before embarking on a course of action. Although the assessment framework varies across professional groups, there are several common principles which should apply in all situations.
- Self-harm means different things to different young people at different times, so the assessment process needs to reflect this. Different types and levels of assessment are needed depending on the context in which professionals work and the severity and complexity of concern about a young person. Options will include referring to more or less specialist assessment services, and professionals must decide whether to assess a young person alone or as part of a wider multi-disciplinary or multi-agency team.
- All young people who have self-harmed should have their psychosocial needs assessed. This is to explore psychological, social and motivational factors that have led to self-harm, as well as to evaluate suicidal intent and the young person's level of hopelessness.
- The assessment process should be extensive, dynamic, and rely on several sources of information from young people, parents or carers, and teachers or other professionals.
- Structured assessment tools can be helpful, but all have their limitations and none predict risk with full certainty. Therefore, they should not be used in isolation or as a substitute for a full assessment, and results of questionnaires or assessment tools should always be considered in context.
- Making sense of the assessment requires the professional to consider the information they have gathered in the context of the research and evidence-based knowledge about self-harm and suicidal behaviour by young people.

Introduction

In order to help young people who self-harm, we must first seek to understand, communicate this understanding and create a therapeutic alliance which is the bedrock for positive change (Armstrong 2006). Assessment is a core part of our work with young people who self-harm, so it is important to be clear about what it means and what it involves. The process of assessing self-harm is as important as any subsequent care or treatment intervention.

This chapter is structured in two parts. First, we explore the component parts of an effective and comprehensive assessment, and second, we describe several standardised assessment tools that can be helpful in assessing self-harming and suicidal young people. Two case vignettes are included to illustrate the common challenges facing professionals who assess self-harming or suicidal young people. The assessment and management of risk, a fundamental part of the overall assessment process, is discussed in a separate chapter.

It is important to say that many young people who self-harm want help, but many resist professional intervention. If they do not want treatment or are unwilling to recognise that their self-harm may be a problem, it will be very difficult to engage them in a meaningful and helpful relationship. As Barish (2004) highlights, a reluctant child is a difficult child to engage. In this case it may be wise to offer brief advice based on safety and harm minimisation followed by the offer that the young person can return for an assessment if they want help and support in the future. This brief intervention may lead to engagement for assessment or treatment at a later date (McKay *et al.* 2006).

Why do an assessment?

Assessment is the decision making process, based upon the collection of relevant information, using a formal set of ethical criteria that contributes to an overall estimation of a person and his circumstances (Barker 2004). It is helpful in understanding how young people perceive, appraise and cope with their difficulties. Assessment is a multifaceted process. It involves asking questions and making observations, both objective and subjective, about how someone looks and behaves and what they are saying to you. Completing a thorough assessment maximises skills of engagement with young people and is more likely to lead to willingness to take up the offer of supportive therapy (Ougrin *et al.* 2009).

A thorough assessment involves the gathering of information from a range of sources and making sense of it. At times, there may be a variance between what a young person says, what they do and what the assessor and others report or observe. All professionals should be expected to make an assessment before embarking on a course of action. Although the assessment framework varies across professional groups, there are several common principles which should apply in all situations. These include the importance of keeping the young person at the centre of care and treatment decisions, using a process which is easy to understand and apply, and not excluding the application of other assessment models.

For many reasons, the assessment of young people who self-harm is often inadequate. The psychosocial and risk assessment of people attending A&E in the UK has been described as lacking, characterised by inadequate inquiry and poor documentation of mental health findings (Merrill *et al.* 1992; Kapur *et al.* 2008; Taylor *et al.* 2009). In undertaking a competent assessment, Brent (1997) suggested the need to cover five domains:

Assessment domains (adapted from Brent 1997)

- Characteristic features of the self-harm attempt
- History of suicidality and psychopathology
- Psychological characteristics
- Family-based factors
- Availability of self-harm means

Similarly, Hawton *et al.* (1982) identified several broad aims of the initial assessment process:

Assessment aims (adapted from Hawton *et al.* 1982)

- Establish a rapport with young person and their family
- Understand reasons for the self-harm
- Clarify the nature of the young person's difficulties
- Identify any possible mental health problems
- Establish what help might be needed

The guidelines proposed by both Brent and Hawton were developed on the basis of extensive clinical experience. How the professional or other adults broker this type of inquiry will vary, but these areas should generally be addressed during the stages of the assessment process.

What kind of assessment?

Arguably, anyone can do an assessment, but what skills does one need in order to perform a 'good' and useful assessment? Engagement through the development of a therapeutic relationship relevant to the context is paramount for two vital reasons. First is about emotional investment. If the young person is not likely to see you again it is important to make this explicit. This helps avoid the young person feeling let down if they expect to receive ongoing support.

Second is about managing expectations. If you plan to work with young people for some time, tell them about the options and how they might want to best use the time. Be clear about your role and remit, are you someone that can 'signpost' them on to a different service, someone who can see them for regular appointments, or someone who they can call to see spontaneously when they feel the need? If you are signposting/referring/transferring them to another service, discuss all the options: Do they want to go there? Would it help if you accompanied them the first time? Could this be part of your role?

Different assessment styles

We saw in Chapter 3 that different professionals use different diagnostic frameworks, formulations and a range of therapeutic models to understand and address self-harming and suicidal behaviour. For example, medical professionals may lean towards the use of psychiatric diagnoses, whereas nurses may be more likely to focus less on the condition and more on how the individual perceives and copes with their difficulties (Altschul 1997). Assessment techniques also vary. Nurses, psychologists and other professionals often use clinical or case formulations, which offer a hypothesis about the cause and nature of the presenting problem.

For example, a psychodynamic formulation will usually comprise a summarising statement, background events and a description of core psychodynamic factors using a specific model and a prognostic assessment (Perry *et al.* 1987). Formulations are considered by some to be less categorical than psychiatric diagnoses (Bond and Bruch 1998). The use of diagnoses, formulations and other conceptual models is often an area of controversy among professionals who work with self-harming or suicidal young people.

Regardless of professional or theoretical orientation, it is essential to apply a systematic framework to assess and understand self-harm. The assessment process will usually lead to a formulation which may or may not include a clinical diagnosis. This is used to base decisions about care planning and management strategies. Again, regardless of one's profession and the assessment tools they use, it is important to keep the young people and, where appropriate, their parents and carers informed about the process.

Assessments in context

Assessments take place in a range of different contexts. Time is often of the essence, and it is important to use the available time a professional has effectively. Sometimes, a snapshot of the key issues will be required whilst other times assessments will be detailed and carried out over a longer period, perhaps during several sessions. The type of assessment needed also depends partly on the seriousness of the situation and who the young person chooses to ask for help. Young people often talk to adults they feel comfortable with, prioritising this over and above the person's knowledge and experience.

In some situations, the health professional is likely to have little prior information on which to base their assessment. In other circumstances it may be possible to perform an assessment which is detailed, comprehensive and based on multiple sources of information. In either case, Mitchell

(2006) suggests that it is important that the health professional performs an assessment that is structured.

Developing a therapeutic relationship

The reaction a young person receives when they reveal their self-harm has a major impact on whether they go on to get help and recover (Jones 2003; Mental Health Foundation and Camelot Foundation 2006). A systematic review conducted by Lambert and Barley (2001) summarised over 100 studies concerning the therapeutic relationship and outcomes of professional intervention. They focused on four areas that influenced service user outcome:

- extra therapeutic factors
- expectancy effects
- specific therapy techniques
- therapeutic relationship factors.

Within the review, the researchers averaged the size of contribution that each predictor made to outcome. They found that 40 per cent of the variance was due to extra therapeutic factors, 15 per cent to expectancy effects, 15 per cent to specific therapy techniques, and 30 per cent of variance was predicted by the therapeutic relationship. Lambert and Barley (2001) concluded that improvement in psychotherapy may best be accomplished by learning to improve ones ability to relate to service users and tailoring that relationship to help meet their needs.

Research findings concerning first responses are important when we consider young people who self-harm. This is in terms of what constitutes good communication skills with children and young people, and an understanding of the predicament the person may be facing (Jones 2003). It has been observed that some children and young people who have had been sexually abused are more sensitive to adult responses, and struggle to communicate their difficulties when asked about them. They may experience fear, embarrassment or feeling that they will not be believed (Lawson and Chaffin 1992; Sharland *et al.* 1996). Whilst we heard earlier that most young people who self-harm have not been sexually abused, a proportion have been. The relationship between sexual abuse and self-harm was discussed in Chapter 2. However, these messages from research may be generally helpful when we consider the overall process of assessment of young people who are often experiencing problems they find difficult to discuss.

Information gathering

Before addressing suicidal or self-harming behaviour, it is important to set the scene by understanding the young person in context. Armstrong (2006) suggests that information about the following factors should be sought:

- family, using family tree or genogram
- peers, school and hobbies
- other agencies and professionals involved
- developmental history
- physical health, emotional health and well-being and history of abuse or neglect
- alcohol or substance misuse
- relationships and support systems
- history of previous self-harm, including knowledge of others that self-harm.

Set in context, an informed assessment also depends on detailed information about the self-harming or suicidal behaviour. This will enable the professional to gain an understanding about issues surrounding the following questions:

- What did the young person do?
- Why did they do it?
- What was their intention?
- How do they feel about it?
- How can the underlying problems be addressed?
- What are their hopes for the future?
- What can be done to change or improve their situation?

For example, when assessing someone after an overdose, we should seek to understand where the tablets were obtained and whether other tablets were taken at the same time. We should seek to establish whether the overdose was impulsive or planned, and if so, how long the young person had been thinking about it. It is also important to know where the young person was when they took their overdose, or if they were in company, who was present. We should ask whether a note or other communication was left which might help clarify motives and intentions.

Corroborating information

Many young people who self-harm have been subjected to numerous assessments by professionals in the various agencies they have come into contact with. Mitchell (2006) reminds us that although assessment of their educational, social care or mental health needs may well have been completed in the past, understanding how such needs impact on the overall functioning of a young person is often lacking. Although previous assessments may be limited in their scope, they may contain important information that will inform decision making in terms of meeting needs and managing risks. Therefore, professionals assessing a young person's self-harming or suicidal behaviour should always seek to obtain and corroborate information from as many sources as possible.

Using several sources of information also generates comparisons, and help clarify inaccuracies or inconsistencies previously not recognised by other professionals. Sometimes these are propagated from one assessment report to another. Mitchell (2006) points out that it is easy to see how myths about needs and risks can be generated and perpetuated. Once in circulation, such myths can easily distort the assessment of needs, risks and negatively influence the service a young person receives as a result (Mitchell 2006).

Assessing the young person

It may seem obvious, but the main ingredient in a thorough assessment is the young person themselves. However, it is often not young people who first ask for help from professionals. Rather, a parent may be worried about their son or daughter's low mood and discuss this with their GP. Alternatively, a school nurse may notice cuts on a student's arm and raise concerns with parents or CAMHS. Whilst the views of parents and others are helpful and inform a valuable part of the assessment, seeing the young person is of utmost importance.

If the young person is happy to be seen on their own, and before seeing their parents, this is ideal as most young people speak more freely when not with others. It is also important not to rush the young person. Studies have shown that assessments that are driven by professionals who dictate the agenda are less effective than those where the pace is led by the young person (Angold 1994). We must, therefore, encourage young people to discuss issues and difficulties as they see them, and at their own pace.

It is important to remember how the assessment process may be perceived by the young people and their parents or carers. Part of forming a therapeutic relationship involves making all those who are involved feel at ease. Talking to young people about general issues can help engage them. Asking what they like and dislike is a way of connecting with people in a manner that is genuine, warm and honest. Young people who self-harm are often sensitive to the appraisal that others may have of them. For this reason, it is important that professionals who offer help are genuine and sincere in their interactions, saying what they mean and meaning what they say (Lewer 2006).

In his book on communicating with vulnerable children and young people, Jones (2003) identifies the following core skills and qualities professionals need to de able to demonstrate effectively:

- listening to the child
- conveying genuine interest
- empathetic concern
- understanding
- emotional warmth
- respect for the child
- capacity to manage and contain the assessment
- awareness of the entire transaction between interviewer and child

- self-management
- technique.

Gender of the professional

The NICE guidelines on self-harm remind us to consider the young person's wishes regarding the gender of the therapist (NICE 2004a). Girls in particular may find it more difficult to talk to a man about certain problems, and there are several reasons for this. It is fine to consider these issues 'out loud' with the young person, giving them options wherever possible. It may be they feel more comfortable having a female present even if they are not able to lead the assessment. In certain contexts, professional trainees can fulfil this role whilst having the dual purpose of enhancing their learning experience.

> What made him think I was going to tell him all my personal stuff when I'd never met him before? He walked in fired questions at me and didn't even seem that interested.
>
> Anne, 16

Creating a climate of safety

Young people who are suicidal or self-harming need to be supported to feel safe during the assessment process. As Lyon (1997) points out, bombarding them with questions will not support a distressed and vulnerable young person who will typically feel powerless and objectified. It is therefore important to set a safe scene. Introductions will include saying 'Hello' to the people present, but also informing them about how long the appointment will last, how things work, and what the overall aims and objectives are. This is in an attempt to make all parties feel as comfortable and involved as possible.

One way to engage young people and their parents or carers can be to do a 'genogram', or family tree. It can also be helpful to talk about friends, school life and hobbies or interests. This enables the person doing the assessment to gain a broad, holistic picture of the person before talking more specifically about their self-harming or suicidal behaviour.

As Professor Phillip Barker reminds us, focusing on people's thoughts, feeling and behaviour are assumed to be human responses to life problems (Barker 2004). The more confident and competent the assessor feels with their role, the more they should be able to make the young person and their family feel at ease. It is important to recognise how hard it may be for a young person to talk about their self-harm. It may take a lot of courage for a person to discuss their thoughts and feelings, and it may be difficult for them to put things into words. Gentle, patient encouragement can help young people feel at ease.

> People don't realise how nervous you can be.
>
> Casey, 16

Most adolescents want to be assessed individually, and for someone to listen to their point of view and try to understand what it is like to be them. However, younger children often feel differently. When given the option to talk on their own or be accompanied by a parent, some will ask for their parent to be present. This is even more likely if the child has never met the professional before. They may be feeling very anxious and fearful about what questions will be asked, and worry what is going to happen to them. It is not unusual for children and adolescents to believe that they will not be allowed home from hospital, that they will be taken into care, or that they or their parents will get into trouble.

> Please explain why you are there and what you are doing and why, so we understand and are not confused, so we feel a little more at ease.
>
> Mia, 13

Meeting with parents and carers

While seeing the young person and talking to them on their own is central to the assessment process, gathering information from others makes the assessment more comprehensive by encompassing other perspectives. Many universal 'Tier 1' CAMHS services, such as school nurses and counsellors, to assess young people on their own. For more specialist assessments, including those undertaken in hospitals or community mental health settings, the involvement of parents and carers is usually required. Typically, the parents or carer of the young person will be invited to accompany the young person and be part of the self-harm assessment process.

Parents and carers can give valuable, additional information by sharing their views on any problems the young person has been having and their ideas about underlying reasons, concerns and possible solutions. Sometimes parents share things that the young person has been worrying about but are unable to say themselves, for example they may be feeling embarrassed about something they have done, such as getting drunk at a party or lying about something at school. Parents may say, did they tell you about 'such and such'. When meeting a professional for the first time, it is not unusual for young people to present a 'good' picture of themselves, so they might leave out certain information that they feel may have a negative influence on the professional.

Developmental history

Depending on the situation and the reasons the young person has self-harmed, it may be important to obtain a detailed developmental history. For instance, their difficulties may have been evident for several years which may point to chronic rather than transient difficulties. The development assessment should include information about the following:

- labour, delivery and birth, including any perinatal complications
- postnatal development, including attachment relationships
- developmental milestones
- temperament
- medical history
- progress at school, including learning difficulties, ability to separate from parents or carers, and comparison to peer group of same age and developmental status.

Significant others

We have heard that the assessment of self-harm and suicidal behaviour often takes place in the hospital setting. If a young person is already known to other professionals, for example a targeted or specialist CAMHS worker, social worker or school counsellor, their views will be an important source of additional assessment information. Likewise, if the young person has already been admitted to hospital, a summary of 'handover' from the nurse in charge of the ward or their key worker is crucial and helpful in making sense of a young person's self-harming behaviour. The following vignette illustrates how this can often be helpful information to consider as part of the overall assessment.

Rachel was observed to be sitting up, eating and drinking normally, smiling and talking to other young people in the paediatric ward. When her mother arrived to visit, Rachel did not speak, lay in bed with covers over her head and refused to eat her lunch.

The physical environment

It is also important to consider the physical environment as this can have an impact on the information obtained during the assessment. Ideally, the room in which a young person is assessed should be inviting, nicely decorated and furnished, enabling young people to feel as comfortable and relaxed as possible. In practice, such ideals can not always be met, and where we assess young people is not always conducive to therapeutic recovery or within our direct control. However, regardless of the environment there are some basic criteria that should always be met.

First, the room should be private. The young person must feel confident that they cannot be overheard by family, friends or strangers. Holding an assessment by the bedside in a hospital ward or in a school corridor does not provide sufficient privacy. Second, wherever possible the assessment should not be interrupted. Some young people find it difficult to articulate how they feel and others are understandably shy, anxious, reticent or mistrustful. If they start talking and are then interrupted by a ringing telephone, call for assistance or other impingement, they may then lose their flow and stop talking. In addition, they might conclude that the person doing the assessment is not fully interested or engaged. It is therefore helpful to put a 'do not disturb' sign on the door and make this clear to colleagues.

The psychological environment

Pacing the assessment and enabling young people to feel comfortable and at ease is a key skill that will help them to express their distress and to share their feelings without getting more anxious. Trust is often a major issue for young people who self-harm, particularly where there are attachment difficulties or there have been previous breaches of trust.

Young people may be wary of what others think about them, or believe professionals and other adults will not understand and that things will be taken out of their control. Edwards (2007) alerts us to the likelihood that trust in a relationship may be regularly tested by young people. They may have lengthy hypothetical discussions about what would happen if they disclosed something, or may test and retest the boundaries of the therapeutic alliance.

Spandler and Warner (2007) emphasise the importance of 'working alongside' young people. This recognises that a young person's self-harm is a coping strategy, and involves reflecting on the therapeutic process rather than jumping to find what might be solutions to eradicate their self-harm, and thus a coping strategy. Giving young people time to explore underlying issues rather than focussing only on the self-harm is crucial. This enables the professional to work in partnership with the young person, and to identify shared goals for the assessment and any subsequent care and treatment.

> I used to think, 'I'm not telling her anything', now I feel I can talk to her about things I couldn't talk to anybody about!
>
> Lauren, 17

If a young person feels engaged with the professional undertaking the assessment they are much more likely to verbalise their thoughts and feelings and share information which will enhance the assessment. Additionally, research has shown time and time again that it is the therapeutic relationship that has most impact on change over and above the choice of therapeutic model delivered. This is discussed in detail in Chapter 7.

Listening

Listening and caring are two of the most important qualities that young people identify as being helpful. It might not seem much, but showing that you want to know and understand can make a positive difference. Active listening is a key assessment skill and is easier said than done. When the professional has heard what the young person has said they then need to check that they have understood it correctly. This clarity can be achieved by paraphrasing or asking the young person whether the key issues they have picked up are the right ones. Clarifying questions such as 'is this what you are saying?', or 'have I understood this correctly?', can be helpful in reaching a shared understanding of the issues and problems facing the young person.

Containment

Working with suicidal or self-harming young people often invokes strong feelings in others, and this is part of human nature. According to psychoanalytic theory, such feelings provide an insight into what the young person may be experiencing, and subsequently what they feel and therefore need. It is important that the professional who is assessing a young person can tolerate and connect with these intense emotions, think about them, attempt to understand them and respond to them. This is the psychodynamic process of containment, and involves a cycle of projection, introjection, reverie and communication (Seinfeld 1996).

> Don't be scared of talking to the person about self-harm or they will get more scared to talk about it too.
>
> Sadie, 15

In providing effective containment for young people who are suicidal or self-harming, it can be helpful to think of what Lewer (2006) calls an 'internal supervisor'. This serves to remind us that the strong emotions we are feeling may be being projected by the young person. If we successfully manage the anxiety that the young person evokes in us, we will signal to them that we can also manage theirs, and trust and development can take place.

If anxiety is not managed, professionals may find themselves tempted to 'do', rather than simply 'be with' young people. This can be a significant obstacle if the young person states that they do not want or need anything from us. If the professional is able to successfully contain strong feelings, the young person is likely to have an experience of being accepted and understood, which assists with engagement and the process of therapy and recovery (Lewer 2006).

Containing anxiety

We have heard that some young people who self-harm go on to kill themselves. It is therefore easy to see how one may become anxious due to the potential risks involved. However, not only does anxiety have a negative effect on our ability to think clearly, but the young people pick up on these feelings. This can feel very uncontaining and may have a negative effect on the engagement process. In contrast, 'holding' – another psychodynamic concept which refers to the ability to contain strong emotions – can enable a suicidal or self-harming young person to feel safe and less overwhelmed.

The self-harming or suicidal behaviour of a young person often arouses huge anxiety in parents, professionals and organisations in which they work. Therefore, containment is an essential skill, not only in terms of working with the young person who self-harms, but also with the systems in which they live and express their needs.

Asking about thoughts and feelings

We have heard that talking to young people about their self-harm does not encourage or make it worse. Importantly, we should explore thoughts and feelings before, during and after the act of self-harm. This is in addition to exploring what the young people did as a result of the thoughts and feelings, and whether other people were involved or alerted as a response. Attitudes towards the self-harm and ideas of regret or remorse are important to identify at this stage.

Good information gathering is assisted by asking general and specific questions. Whilst some young people appear to find structured questions confrontational and difficult to answer, others find them easier than a less systematic method of enquiry:

> It's easier when you're asked specific questions, instead of just being expected to talk and you don't know what to say – then you can tell them what they want to know.
>
> Casey, 16

However it shouldn't feel too formal or one-sided either:

> It's better when it feels like a conversation rather than an interview.
>
> Holly, 17

We need to keep in mind that young people don't always have the answers to questions we may ask:

> You can feel pressured when you are asked certain questions such as, 'why do you self-harm?' when you are not sure yourself!
>
> Lauren, 17

The importance of non-verbal communication

So far, we have considered the ways in which professionals can gather information through questioning and corroborating information from third parties. However, it is also important to consider non-verbal communications and whether they give the same or different impressions when compared to verbal or written accounts.

For example, a young person might say that they feel calm when they look quite agitated. Alternatively, a young person may say they feel fine when they are clearly upset. Non-verbal communications include facial expressions (including eye contact), as well as posture, gestures and other behaviours. For suicidal young people, it is especially important to be aware of both verbal and non-verbal communication, as what they say might not always reflect how they feel and what they are planning to do.

Mental health assessment

A comprehensive self-harm assessment should also include a focus on mental health and disorder. This is to identify symptoms of known risk factors for self-harm and suicidal behaviour, including depression and psychosis.

Assessing mood

Descriptions of the young person's mood over recent weeks can tell us a lot about how they are feeling and if this changes in different circumstances. It is useful to know if there are times when the young person feels happy and looks forward to things, has a sense of self-worth and enjoyment, as well as gaining an understanding about episodes of low or depressed mood.

Some young people will describe how they are fine at school and when out with friends, but once they return home their mood changes and they feel depressed. Others experience the opposite and struggle more at school and in social situations. If young people use the term 'depression', it is important to explore what they mean. As well as a commonly used word, which can be used in a different ways that may not be the same, depression is also a common mental disorder. The term 'depression' may be a euphemism for feeling sad, upset or unhappy in given circumstances, or it may be associated with a clinical disorder, the symptoms of which are described below.

Common symptoms of depression

- Persistent low mood, unhappiness and irritability
- Loss of interest in recreation, activity and friends
- Loss of energy and concentration
- Deterioration in school or work performance
- Change in appetite with corresponding weight change
- Disturbed sleep
- Thoughts of worthlessness and suicide
- Somatic complaints, e.g. headache, abdominal pain

If a young person's low mood continues for several weeks and seems pervasive in all situations, then it may be helpful to refer the young person for a specialist, comprehensive mental health assessment, and they may require psychological and/or pharmacological treatment. The NICE guidelines on depression in children and young people (National Collaborating Centre for Mental Health 2005) give comprehensive information about the roles and responsibilities of all professionals who work with children and young people.

It is important to note that some young people can present with quite vague symptoms, seeking out help without a clear idea or understanding of what they feel is wrong. This situation can be quite challenging for professionals who may be faced with a dilemma. On the one hand, due to the risks involved, it is imperative that symptoms of mental disorder are not missed or left untreated. On the other, there may be concern about the issue of 'pathologising' or the unhelpful labelling of young people who are arguably reacting normally, albeit in self-destructive ways, to adverse life events.

If a professional or other adult has concerns about a young person's low mood, it is reasonable to discuss these with the young person and their family. Some people find a name or label for symptoms of depression helpful whereas others find them unhelpful and stigmatising. Importantly, whatever the feelings of low mood are called, it is important to address these and seek ways in which young people can be supported to feel better. For professionals who are not trained to recognise depression, it is important that reports of symptoms listed earlier are discussed with specialist CAMHS colleagues (de Wilde *et al.* 2001).

> I told my GP how I was feeling low and he wanted to put me on anti-depressants. I didn't want to take tablets. I wanted to sort out the problems.
>
> Lisa, 17

Other mental health problems

Whilst suicidal ideation in adolescence is most strongly associated with depression, other disorders, such as anxiety, psychosis and substance misuse can also exist (Lewinsohn *et al.* 1996; Hawton *et al.* 2005). The mental health assessment, therefore, needs to include consideration of broader mental health issues, including phobias, compulsions or anxiety, eating disorders, substance misuse, and bipolar and attention deficit hyperactivity disorder (ADHD).

Any feelings of hope and hopelessness that are expressed by young people also need to be explored. This can be done using narrative, where the young person gives an account of how they see their future, or it can be addressed by using a 'scaling question'. For example, we often ask a young person how hopeful they feel about the future on a scale of one to ten. However, it is important to be clear whether the number zero or ten is as bad as it could get.

It can be reassuring and protective if, whilst a young person is very distressed, they also remain hopeful about their future. Questions and observation in relation to appearance and self-care, eye contact, agitation, speech, mood, concentration, self-image and insight to their problems also help elicit useful information that contributes to an overall picture of a young person's mental state.

Structured assessment tools

A range of structured assessment tools and screening instruments are available which may be helpful when assessing self-harm and suicide. Some of these are general and address related issues such as depression or risk factors. Others are specific and focus on self-harm or suicidal behaviour, and these are discussed in the next chapter. Some of those that focus on general functioning and issues commonly related to self-harm are listed below.

Beck Hopelessness Scale

The Beck Hopelessness Scale (BHS) is a brief self-report inventory. There are 20 items assessing feelings about the future, loss of motivation and expectations. Each item consists of a 'true or false' statement and is scored zero or one. Negative responses on each item are added together to give a total score out of 20. The BHS is designed for use with people aged over 17. The Hopelessness

Scale for Children (HSC) is a 17-item scale used with children aged 6–13 and has been adapted from the BHS.

Beck Depression Inventory

The Beck Hopelessness Scale correlates with the Beck Depression Inventory (BDI, BDI-II) and the two are commonly used in conjunction. Suitable for children and young people aged over 13, the BDI is a multiple-choice self-report inventory. It includes questions on cognitive processes, such as guilt, hopeless and irritability, as well as physical symptoms of depression, such as loss of weight, tiredness and apathy. There are three versions of the BDI. The original was first published in 1961 and was revised in 1978 as the BDI-1A. More recently the BDI-II was published and is used by health professionals and researchers.

Like many self-rating tools, the scores can either be minimised or exaggerated by young people who complete them. This means that results must always be considered in the context of the wider assessment.

Hospital Anxiety and Depression Rating Scale

The Hospital Anxiety and Depression Rating Scale (HADS) (Zigmund and Snaith 1983) is a commonly used screening and self-rating questionnaire. It can be used with adolescents and young people in a range of settings, and only takes a few minutes to complete.

HoNOSCA

The Health of the Nation Outcome Scale for Children and Adolescents (HoNOSCA) is a routine outcome measurement tool which assesses the behaviours, impairments, symptoms and social functioning of children and adolescents with mental health problems (Gowers *et al.* 1998). There are separate versions for clinician use and for parents and young people to complete. HoNOSCA scales cover a number of domains, including non-accidental self-injury and raters are asked to report self-harm such as hitting self, self-cutting, suicide attempts, overdoses, hanging and drowning. Self-harm behaviour is rated on a scale of 0–4:

0   No problem of this kind during the period rated.
1   Occasional thoughts about death or of self-harm not leading to injury. No self-harm or suicidal thoughts.
2   Non-hazardous self-harm such as wrist scratching, whether or not associated with suicidal thoughts.
3   Moderately severe suicidal intent (including preparatory acts e.g. collecting tablets) or moderate non-hazardous self-harm (e.g. small overdose).
4   Serious suicidal attempt (e.g. serious overdose), or serious deliberate self-injury.

Strengths and Difficulties Questionnaire

The Strengths and Difficulties Questionnaire (SDQ) (Goodman 1997) is a brief behavioural screening questionnaire for children and adolescents aged 4–16. Several versions exist which have been adapted to suit the needs of clinicians and researchers. Although the SDQ does not address self-harm directly, it covers many areas which young people may be struggling with on a day-to-day basis.

Children's Global Assessment Scale

The Children's Global Assessment Scale (CGAS) (Shaffer *et al.* 1983) is a numeric scale (1–100) used by mental health professionals to rate the general functioning of children and young people under the age of 18. It does not directly address self-harm, but provides anchor point descriptions of behavioural functioning.

Salford Needs Assessment Schedule for Adolescents

The Salford Needs Assessment Schedule for Adolescents (SNASA) (Kroll *et al.* 1999) is a generalised needs assessment measure for use with young people. It is comprehensive and addresses multiple domains of need. Outcomes are generated from current and historical information provided by the young person and their parent, carer or other significant adult.

What are the limitations of assessment tools?

The use of structured assessment tools, particularly those that have been researched, developed and validated in clinical practice, inform decisions about the most effective way to meet the young person's needs (Mitchell 2006). However, for any assessment tool to be used effectively, it is important that the professional administering the tool has been trained to use it. They must also be aware of the specific strengths and weaknesses of the particular assessment tool.

Mitchell (2006) suggests that assessment tools do not disempower the health professional or stifle individual clinical judgement. Rather, he proposes where an assessment tool produces an outcome that the professional considers to be unrealistic, it is important that clinical judgement and discussion with the multi-disciplinary team is factored into the evaluation and outcome process of assessment. It is the combination of an experienced professional using a structured, validated tool which is likely to produce the best outcomes whether it is needs or risk that are being assessed (Mitchell 2006).

Some assessments may involve asking a few simple questions, but when the assessment concerns a young person who has self-harmed and may be at risk of suicide, professionals may need to use a more comprehensive and dynamic assessment process. For this purpose, many professionals and services choose to adopt or design an assessment proforma such as the one used by

Nottingham CAMHS self-harm team (see Table 5.1). These can be extremely helpful in reminding us to address all important areas and reduce the chances of missing key information.

The Nottingham self-harm pro forma is useful for those who may be less familiar and confident about assessing a young person who has self-harmed. In some situations it is acceptable to allow the assessment to be led by the young person and further information can be gathered at a subsequent appointment. However, when assessing self-harm and suicidal intent, missing key information could lead to a fatal outcome, so the assessment should always be structured. Like all human beings, health professionals perform better some days than others, and errors do occur. Having the support and structure of a framework such as the Nottingham self-harm pro forma leaves less to memory and helps to reduce omissions which may lead to potentially fatal consequences.

It is important to point out that the pro forma is a guide, it is not intended to be 'read out' word for word and, where relevant, questions should be expanded and more detail obtained. The themes on the pro forma are selected from a contemporary evidence base, and regularly reviewed, ensuring that key questions are asked, which would include information about both risk and needs as recommended by NICE (2004a).

Table 5.1 Nottingham self-harm pro forma

Care Pathway standards for Young People under 16 admitted to medical wards (and all ages on paediatric wards) following attendance at Emergency Department for episode of self-harm. Young people should be referred to CAMHS when medically and physically fit.

Intervention	Date/ Initial	Tick and explain N/A and No
Choice of therapist gender discussed		[ ] Yes [ ] No
Request for specific therapist gender available		[ ] Yes – state [ ] No [ ] N/A
CAMHS self-harm risk and needs assessment form completed – enclosed in notes		[ ] Yes [ ] No [ ] N/A
Young person seen alone (without parent)		[ ] Yes [ ] No [ ] N/A
Parent/carer present for part of assessment		[ ] Yes [ ] No [ ] N/A
Management plan completed – in notes		[ ] Yes [ ] No [ ] N/A

Table 5.1 continued

Intervention	Date/ Initial	Tick and explain N/A and No
Young person contributed to/agreement with management plan		[ ] Yes [ ] No [ ] N/A
Parent/carer contributed to/agreement with management plan		[ ] Yes [ ] No [ ] N/A
Copy of management plan given to young person/ parent/carer		[ ] Yes [ ] No [ ] N/A
Recognised CAMHS risk assessment completed		[ ] SH assessment form [ ] Level 1 – green sheet [ ] Level 2 – CPA [ ] FACE
Assessed for CPA		[ ] Yes [ ] No [ ] N/A
Care plan/CPA process completed		[ ] Yes [ ] No [ ] N/A
Discussed concerns/advice sought from colleague		[ ] Psychiatrist [ ] Other MDT – state [ ] No
Use of rating scales		[ ] Yes – state which one/s? [ ] No
CAMHS outcome measures completed		[ ] HoNOSCA [ ] SDQ [ ] CHI-ESQ [ ] CGAS [ ] CORC
Information given to service user		[ ] Choice leaflet [ ] YP self-harm leaflet [ ] Parent/carer self-harm leaflet [ ] Getting involved with CAMHS [ ] YP – feedback forms [ ] Parent/carer – feedback forms
Discussed young person in clinical supervision		[ ] Yes [ ] No [ ] N/A
Received follow-up appointment within 14 days		[ ] Yes [ ] No [ ] N/A

Young people in complex situations

Sometimes an assessment is fairly straightforward. The young person and the family are engaged in the process, they agree about the precipitating circumstances, the young person regrets what they have done, the family is supportive and there is a clear agreed plan about how to help things improve. However, at other times the process is less straightforward.

Young people who self-harm are not always easy to engage, and of course some choose to decline the offer of support. For those that do agree to have an assessment and then don't show up at the hospital or clinic setting, a home visit may need to be arranged. Some young people may even resort to locking themselves in their bedroom and refuse to talk or come out. Here, the professional needs to consider whether the young person is at risk and whether the young person is able to decide for themselves whether they need to be assessed. This depends on a range of issues including age, competence, risk and resilience factors.

If an assessment is difficult to conduct because the young person is reluctant to engage with the process, then the professional must prioritise what they need to achieve. If a full assessment is not possible, then it is important to establish the meaning of the self-harm, specifically if it is done with any suicidal intent. Often, the self-harming or suicidal young person is not known to professional services and is first encountered in a crisis situation. Here, it is essential that the professional undertaking the assessment gathers as much information as possible about the precipitating factors, antecedents and self-harming behaviour itself. In these circumstances, the assessment of risk is crucially important.

Matthew

Matthew, aged 14, presents at A&E saying he has taken an undisclosed number of tablets. The nurse who assesses Matthew has met him previously and is not convinced. She arranges for Matthew to have a blood test to be on the safe side. His blood results indicate that very low levels of paracetamol are present and this is not consistent with his reports of an overdose. The nurse notes from Matthew's records that he has presented at A&E on five separate occasions in the last month saying the same thing. Each time, his blood results do not corroborate his overdose claims. How can this situation best be managed?

Difficult decisions

As Matthew's case illustrates, there are circumstances in which a young person self-harms that may challenge our ethical values, codes and preferences. If a young person tells you they have taken an overdose, then they need to get urgent medical attention. National guidance indicates that all young people under 16 years old should be admitted to a hospital medical ward for a comprehensive self-harm assessment from a specialist CAMHS team. If a young person has cut or burned themselves it will depend on the severity, frequency, their intentions and involvement with services as to whether they need to attend hospital for a specialist CAMHS assessment (Royal College of Psychiatrists 1998; 2004b).

In Matthew's situation, it is best not to share our thoughts and doubts with him. Fearing that he is not to be believed or taken seriously may lead Matthew to feel rejected. He may then feel angry, guilty or upset and then take a 'real' overdose. It is generally better to be safe than sorry. Treating someone who says they have taken an overdose and may not have done, is less potentially harmful than challenging them in a way they may not be able to cope with, thus increasing the risks. In this situation, it would be sensible for the nurse assessing Matthew to discuss the situation and circumstances with her colleagues. Together, they may consider that it is not appropriate, or 'safe enough', to share their reticence about Matthew's alleged overdose directly with him.

However, it may be appropriate to address this issue at a point when Matthew is feeling safer and is not in a crisis situation. A good therapeutic relationship may have formed, and it may be possible to encourage Matthew to talk about his worries and concerns, and the reasons he feels the need to present to crisis services saying he has taken an overdose. Reflecting together that taking tablets, or saying you have, will not resolve the problems, but in fact create some additional ones, may be helpful in identifying opportunities for positive change. However, conversations of this nature should always be conducted with sensitivity and understanding, rather than challenge or confrontation.

Usually asking questions and inviting curiosity leads to further understanding of a situation. But again, there are times when we would choose not to be curious, not to ask further questions, and not want to expand. This is not to show disinterest, but is to address the critical issues before returning to motives and curiosity. The importance of avoiding challenge and confrontation is illustrated in Rochelle's case:

Rochelle

Rochelle says she took an overdose of ten parcetamol tablets because she wanted to die. She took the tablets while travelling home on the school bus. Her best friend Kate took the tablets from Rochelle to prevent her taking any more. Rochelle is unknown to services.

Health professionals are often asked to assess a suicidal or self-harming young person for the first time. They have not yet got to know them, which makes it difficult to draw conclusions about their behaviour. In this situation, it would not be appropriate to take risks and challenge Rochelle's motivation. It would not be helpful to say that she would be unlikely to die taking tablets in front of her friends. Rather, it would be important to connect to how she was feeling and to try and understand what led her to behave in this way.

Sometimes it is parents who are expressing doubts and are not sure how to handle the situation. Parents sometimes doubt the suicidal intent of their son or daughter who is expressing a wish to die, or may suggest that claims of self-harm are exaggerated or made up. Again, it is often best not to challenge at the stage where emotions may be running high and the family are distressed and vulnerable. A discussion could take place at a later time, if that feels right, or it may be that the situation is never discussed or clarified.

What do young people tell us about assessment?

The following list of helpful and unhelpful interventions for assessment was created by young people in a repeat self-harm group in Nottingham (see Table 5.2).

Making sense of the assessment information – informed judgements

So far we have discussed how to use engagement and assessment skills to gather as much relevant information as possible within the time available in any given context or circumstance. This is then applied to what we understand about research and evidence-based practice about self-harm and suicidal behaviour by young people.

Often, a decision will need to be made about whether to make a referral to another service. This may be for more specialist assessment and intervention, or for a service more 'accessible' to the young person in terms of location and possible appeal or attraction. It is important to give the young person some choice as a way of encouraging them to seek help, and they may perceive some services as less stigmatising than others.

Table 5.2 Dos and don'ts of assessment (Nottingham repeat self-harm group)

DO	DON'T
Act like a friend, be friendly	Judge me and patronise me
Make me feel comfortable	Ask 'how does that make you feel'?
Talk to me and see me as a 'whole' person	Avoid talking about self-harm or suicidal feelings
Make me feel like you care	Be scared of self-harm
Talk about self-harm	Just talk about self-harm

Summary

With appropriate education, training, support and supervision most professionals can undertake assessments of young people who self-harm (Wright and Richardson 2003). We have discussed what an assessment is, why it is needed and what to include, considered aspects of how to conduct an assessment and tools that may be used to facilitate the process. We have put this in the context of adolescent development which is an evolving process.

Self-harm means different things to different young people at different times and so the assessment process needs to reflect this. Different types and levels of assessment are needed depending on the context in which professionals work and the severity and complexity of concern about a young person.

Options will include referring to more or less specialist assessment services, and professionals must decide whether to assess a young person alone or as part of a wider assessment team. The assessment and management of risk is part and parcel of the overall assessment process, and is discussed in the next chapter.

6   Assessing and managing the risk of self-harm and suicide

Key points:

- All young people who have self-harmed should have their risk assessed as part of a broader psychosocial assessment. The risk assessment should focus on triggers and the severity of the self-harm, and maintaining factors which may lead to repetition.
- Assessing suicidal intent is a key part of the assessment process and it is often inadequate. Young people who repeatedly self-harm do not always do so for the same reason and by the same means, making evaluation of motivation and intent a challenging process.
- A focus on impulsivity and planning is crucial. It is important to establish whether steps were taken to avoid discovery, or if preparations for death were made. A tendency to impulsive behaviour may increase risk of repetition, but it is important to remember that an impulsive act can be just as damaging or potentially fatal as a planned one.
- There are a number of known risk factors to consider when making sense of assessment information. These may increase the likelihood of further self-harming or suicidal behaviour.
- Just as it is crucial to assess risk, so too is it important to assess protective factors, strengths and resources in the young person, family and wider community network. This is to inform decisions about whether the risks and benefits of professional intervention outweigh the risks of non-intervention.
- Risk management entails finding the best possible solution to a given problem. It involves consideration of all the options, eliminating the ones that are less helpful, and selecting those that are most suitable.

Introduction

All professionals who work with children and young people share a duty to keep them safe (Department for Education and Skills 2003). Recognising and reducing the potential risk of self-harm, suicide and self-neglect is central to our work, and this is with the fundamental aim of improving quality of life and promoting recovery. In essence, the better our knowledge about a young person, the better our risk assessment is likely to be.

Just as it is crucial to assess risk, so too is it important to assess strengths and protective factors in the young person, family and wider community network. This is to inform decisions about whether the risks and benefits of professional intervention outweigh the risks of non-intervention (Ryan and McDougall 2008).

What is risk?

Risk refers to the factors in a child or young person's life that may have a negative impact on their health, development and psychosocial functioning. It is important for us to distinguish between acute and chronic risks. We have previously heard that self-harm and suicidal behaviours occur for a variety of reasons. Among other things, this includes managing strong negative emotions, to elicit care from someone, to cope with dissociation, or to end one's life.

Acute risks are those which occur in the context of crisis and further increase the likelihood of suicidal behaviour. In contrast, chronic risk refers to the long-term risk of self-harm and suicide. A 2009 poll by YoungMinds asked children and young people about the difficulties they experienced which could be regarded as risks.

Problems that concern children

- Bullying
- Siblings being mean
- Parents getting divorced
- Family problems
- Living with parents who don't look after you
- Fears about being taken away from your parents
- Worries about money
- Someone hurting your body
- Mum and Dad always arguing
- Missing friends
- Relationship problems
- Drugs and alcohol
- Isolation
- Boredom
- Things that we see in the news that no-one talks to us properly about

YoundMinds 2009

Raby and Raby (2008) warn that risks can have a domino effect, that is, where one problem can lead to the development of a series of other problems.

How do we assess risk?

Risk assessment is an examination of the context and the detail of past risk incidents, in the light of current circumstances. From this we can extrapolate predictions of the future likelihood of risk behaviours (Morgan 2003). This, of course, is not an exact science and it is not possible to predict which young people will kill themselves (Hargus *et al.* 2009).

Assessment of levels of risk and predictions of future risk are difficult to quantify with accuracy; they are guides, not absolutes, established with the information available at that specific time. The Department of Health (2007b) gives comprehensive guidance and identifies best practice for understanding, assessing and managing risk. It suggests that a thorough risk assessment should focus on the following three questions:

- how likely is it that the event will occur?
- how soon is it expected to occur?
- how severe will the outcome be if it does occur?

According to the NICE guidelines an assessment of self-harm should focus both on risk and on needs (NICE 2004a). The assessment of suicidal risk is undoubtedly the most important part of a self-harm treatment package and it is often inadequate (Sheldrick 1999). A risk and needs assessment is a dynamic, ongoing process. Changes can occur at any time, making the situation likely to be more or less risky, so the process needs to be continually reviewed. Mitchell (2006) states that risk assessment and risk management should be considered as two sides of the same coin. It is pointless to undertake an assessment of risk unless consideration is given as to how that risk will be managed.

Assessing suicidal thoughts

When young people tell us they are feeling suicidal or have thoughts of wanting to die, we need to take this very seriously and talk with them in detail. Suicidal thoughts and their association with self-harming or suicidal behaviour can range in intensity from:

- expressions to self or out loud to others – without real conviction or intent;
- vague, passive feelings of wishing one was better off dead;
- thoughts that lead to self-harm in a safe context where outcomes are largely known;
- thoughts that lead to self-harm in an unsafe context where outcomes are largely unknown; and
- thoughts leading to self-harm likely to cause significant harm or be fatal.

According to O'Driscoll and Holden (2002), suicidal intentions and help seeking behaviours may be expressed in a variety of ways including:

- overt verbal or written expression of suicidal thoughts, preparations or plans;
- definite statements of intent, for example; 'I've had enough, I want to kill myself';
- vague or suggestive statements of intent, for example; 'Don't bother with me', 'I'm more trouble than I'm worth', or 'People would be better off without me';
- non-verbal indications, such as uncharacteristic increased or decreased contact with care staff;
- metaphorical statements of intent, for example getting one's affairs in order, saying goodbye, giving away belongings, or returning borrowed items.

Although guidance for professionals on assessing risk following self-harm by adults is available (Royal College of Psychiatrists (2004b), there are fewer resources that focus on risk assessment in children and young people. Hawton and Rodham (2006a) propose that instruments that have been used to evaluate suicidal behaviours in children and adolescents can be divided into those that assess:

- the presence of suicidal behaviours
- the risk or propensity for suicidal behaviours
- the intentionality and medial lethality of suicidal behaviours
- exposure to suicidal behaviour.

Known risk factors

There are a number of known risk factors to consider when making sense of assessment information. The following factors increase the likelihood of further self-harm, and have been derived from research.

- Gender – male (suicide); female (self-harm) (Madge 1996)
- Previous self-harm (Gunnell *et al.* 2008)
- Mental health problems e.g. depression (Beautrais *et al.* 1998; Beautrais 2001)
- Hopelessness or lack of goals (Beck *et al.* 1993; Marciano and Kazdin 1994; Kerfoot *et al.* 1996)
- Impulsiveness (Kingsbury *et al.* 1999; Evans *et al.* 1996)
- Lack of support from family and friends, social isolation (Morano *et al.* 1993)

- Bullying (NSPCC 2008a)
- Poor coping/problem solving ability (Schotte and Clum 1987; Speckens and Hawton 2005; McAuliffe *et al.* 2006)
- History of abuse (Kendall-Tackett *et al.* 1993)
- Substance misuse (Rossow *et al.* 2009)
- Unemployment (Young *et al.* 2007)
- Access to self-harm means

Research by Sankey and Lawrence (2005) put some of these risk factors into context. They studied case records of suicides and risk-taking deaths in 12–17-year-olds in New South Wales and found three distinct groups:

1   Sixty-six per cent had enduring difficulties based within the family, mental health and school.
2   Fourteen per cent had recently experienced a pivotal life event including relationship break-ups, deaths or a major argument.
3   Fifteen per cent had experimented with drugs.

Previously Shaffer (1974) has suggested there were two types of children who kill themselves:

1   highly intelligent, socially isolated with mentally ill mothers
2   aggressive, impulsive and often in trouble at school.

In their excellent book, Hawton and Rodham (2006b) reflected on the reasons 6,000 young people gave for their experiences of self-harm or suicidal behaviour. This includes a focus on the risk and protective factors for self-harm, and professionals are offered guidance on how to recognise those who may be at greatest risk.

Regardless of the event experienced and what may appear trivial to an adult, it is important that professionals are mindful that problems may seem insurmountable to an adolescent. Just as it is not only the quantity of tablets that a young person has taken, but their understanding of lethality that informs risk – it is not the severity of the event that has occurred, but a young person's perception of severity which is important. Matching these factors to the information gained, along with knowledge about protective factors, helps us make a formulation and subsequent risk management plan.

Ambivalence

Self-harm and suicidal behaviour is often accompanied by ambivalence. Young people may have thoughts of wanting to kill themselves with varying degrees of commitment to carry out these ideas. This may vary from vague feelings, to ambivalence, to definite plans. Suicidal thoughts can also change quickly and are likely to be more or less intense depending on the levels of stress a young person may be experiencing.

In addition, what starts off as suicidal behaviour for some young people may evolve over time to become non-suicidal behaviour. In contrast, young people may have completed suicide when death was not their intention, that is, where their actions were by accident as opposed to design.

Furthermore, we need to be aware that what young people say and tell us and what they have done are not always the same. Sometimes young people want us to believe they have made a serious suicide attempt, when they have not, perhaps to get us to understand how they are feeling about the situation they find themselves in and to get some help.

More worryingly, others may tell us that they are coping and try to convince us that all is well. They may be telling us what they think we want to hear to reduce our levels of concern. This may be with the intention of putting plans to kill themselves into action. It goes without saying that professionals should be mindful of this scenario in every self-harm risk assessment.

Adolescent errors of judgement

We saw earlier in the book that risk-taking behaviour during adolescence can be seen as part of identity formation and, to some extent, a normal developmental task. Research by Rodham and colleagues (2006b) has focused on adolescents' perceptions of risk, and found that they perceive risk as something where the outcome is uncontrollable. This is compared to a challenge where there is a known end point, even though it might be difficult to achieve.

The study showed that adolescents were confident in their ability to make rational decisions having weighed up the pros and cons and had an overall appreciation of risks. However, there was some evidence to suggest that their lack of knowledge and life experience may lead to errors of judgement. Rodham *et al.* went on to suggest that some adolescents lack the ability to assertively state when they do not want to engage in a particular behaviour for fear of peer rejection. This clearly impacts negatively when the behaviour involves harm to self.

An example of this is a young person who miscalculated the risk of taking an overdose of 30 tablets.

Rachel

Rachel took 30 paracetamol knowing that she would be OK. She 'knew' this because her friend Sarah had taken more than this a few times and Sarah was OK.

Rachel's overdose was perceived as a serious risk by her concerned parents and other adults, but based on her friend Sarah's overdoses, Rachel did not believe that she would come to harm. This, of course, is an error of judgement. Just because one adolescent tolerated 30 tablets without evidently suffering serious harm, this does not mean than another person's body would react in the same way. Indeed, very small overdoses of paracetamol have proven to be lethal, whereas, on other occasions, larger overdoses have not resulted in permanent damage or death.

Another illustration of how adolescents may misjudge the anticipated response to their self-harming behaviour is illustrated in the following vignette:

Tom

Tom took an overdose of tablets 'safe' in the knowledge that his mother would see the empty packet when she returned from work.

Tom took a controlled overdose as a way of asking for help, but presumed that a number of factors that were actually beyond his control would be predictable. Indeed, Tom's mother might have been late returning from work, or fail to notice the empty packet of tablets. She may even have chosen to conclude herself that Tom had taken a 'safe' overdose based on her previous experience of managing Tom in this situation. These are dynamic factors which Tom may not have fully considered and which may have delayed access to urgent medical attention.

It is therefore essential to explore beliefs about self-harming behaviour as part of the risk assessment process. It is common for young people to underestimate the severity of their self-harming behaviour. They may be ill informed about the associated problems which may include mental and physical health problems, school exclusion and the risk of death.

Concerns about immediate risk – suicide and safety

The fundamental aim of a self-harm assessment is to keep the young person safe. The evaluation of risk should primarily be organised around a central question – is this young person able to keep themselves safe? The previous chapter shows that answering this question competently depends on engaging the young person first. The following vignette illustrates the issues to be considered:

Stacey

Stacey, aged 13, took an overdose of yew tree berries. She subsequently suffered a cardiac arrest. Her parents are distraught and cannot understand why their daughter is feeling so bad. Stacey is not sure why she took the yew tree berries and isn't sure whether she wanted to die. She is assessed on a cardiac ward with her parents present.

Armstrong suggests how judgements about risk may be formulated:

- How much substance was accessible/available/taken?
- Were drugs or alcohol involved? If so, which drugs or alcohol and how much?
- Was the overdose planned or impulsive?
- Was the overdose taken whilst the young person was alone? If not, who was present?
- Were active precautions taken to avoid discovery?
- How much does the young person know about the lethality/harmful effects of the overdose?
- Was a suicide note written?
- Did the young person tell anyone before or after the overdose?
- Did the young person attempt to gain help during or after the overdose?
- Is the young person regretful or disappointed to be alive?
- Would the young person take another overdose?
- Is the young person planning to take another overdose?
- How hopeful/hopeless does the young person feel about the future?

(Armstrong 2006)

If the professional undertaking the assessment is concerned that a young person is imminently at risk of suicide, then an action plan needs to be developed and implemented. The young person and their parents or carers may have ideas about how to keep the young person safe until the acute crisis is resolved. For instance, this might involve not having to see particular people, seeing others, having some time out, staying with a supportive family member, or not spending time alone. The ability of parents or carers to keep their son or daughter safe should be part of the overall assessment process.

Is it safe for the young person to be at home?

Risk management entails finding the best possible solution to a given problem. It involves consideration of all the options, eliminating the ones that are less helpful, and selecting those that are most suitable. For the large majority of young people who self-harm this will mean remaining at home with their parents or carers. In some circumstances, the risks may be so high that admission to hospital or another residential setting may be required. However, this can bring additional risks associated with social contagion, which were discussed earlier in the book.

The purpose of inpatient adolescent mental health units is primarily for the assessment and treatment of young people with severe mental health problems. Many young people who self-harm do not fit this description, so it is only in rare circumstances when the person is considered to be at imminent risk of suicide that admission should be considered.

If a young person is struggling with chronic life stresses and these are likely to continue, then a short stay on an adolescent unit is unlikely to change this situation. Professionals therefore need to find a way to support the young person and the family, and this will often mean multi-agency partnership working to develop an agreed management plan. In rare circumstances, the young person may be accommodated in local authority secure facilities if their safety cannot be managed at home or in an alternative community setting.

Whilst some people may come into hospital as a place of safety, with the hope of getting help, it is important to note that for some their intention is to kill themselves. If their suicidal thoughts have led them to make detailed plans, they may view it as a neutral place, or as being less painful to their family. The multi-disciplinary team needs to keep this possibility in mind.

Risk assessment tools

We saw in the previous chapter that all assessment tools have their limitations in terms of scope and validity. This is pertinent when we consider risk because no assessment tools predict risk with full certainty. This is because the absolute risk of suicide is very low (Dennehy *et al.* 1996).

Most of the available risk assessment tools come from the US (Fox and Hawton 2004). They are imprecise in that they sometimes overestimate (false positives) or underestimate (false negatives) needs or risks. Therefore, risk assessment measures should not be used in isolation or as a substitute for a full assessment, and results of questionnaires or assessment tools should always be considered in context. Nor should risk assessment measures be used to justify not offering or withholding a service to a young person considered to be low risk. As Lyon (1997) puts it, no checklist can spell away the real fears of a distressed young person or their worker.

A number of resources have been developed to assist professionals and other adults who work with young people who self-harm in providing safe and competent interventions. The following risk assessment tools and resources may be helpful as part of a wider assessment of self-harming or suicidal young people.

Pierce Suicidal Intent Scale

This interview-based or self-administered scale is derived from the Beck Scales and is designed to assess the intention to die among people who have attempted suicide (Pierce 1997). It has 15 items separated into circumstances related to the suicide attempt (e.g. presence of a suicide note) and self-report items (e.g. expectations of fatality). The first group of items can be completed retrospectively from case notes. Each item is scored on a three-point scale and cut-offs for severity are provided. Five additional items do not contribute to the overall score. There are no specific cut-offs and a positive response to any item should be a cause for concern for professionals. Although the Suicidal

Intent Scale is used widely, there has been a lack of research focusing on its use with young people (Antretter *et al.* 2008).

Scale for Suicide Ideation

Again based on original Beck Scales, the Beck Scale for Suicide Ideation (BSS) assesses an individual's thoughts, attitudes and intentions about suicide. This is a 21-item scale which can be completed by a practitioner or the young person themselves. The BSS is designed to assess the intensity of a person's attitudes towards suicide, as well as their behaviours and plans to complete suicide during the past week. Some 19 test items are each rated between zero and two and added together to yield a total score ranging from 0–38. Two additional items ask about previous suicide attempts and the seriousness of intent during the most recent episode. The first five of the 19 items act as a screening filter. Whilst a higher score is associated with a higher risk, there are no specific cut-offs. As with the Pierce scale, a positive response to any item should concern professionals.

SAD PERSONS

The SAD PERSONS Scale is a suicide risk scale to assess immediate probability of suicidal behaviours. The scale's name is an acronym, with each letter representing one of the ten risk factors that are identified. Although the scale has been found to provide a semi-structured framework for the assessment process, it lacks reliability and validity measures (Juhnke 1994).

The SAD PERSONS Scale has been adapted for use with children and young people (A-SPS). The specific risk factors addressed in the scale are: age; depression or affective disorder; previous attempt; alcohol or drug abuse; rational thinking loss; social supports lacking; organised plan; negligent parenting; significant family stressors; suicidal modelling by parents or siblings; and problems at school (Juhnke 1996).

PATHOS

PATHOS is a screening questionnaire which is used to identify young people aged 13–18 who are at high risk after taking an overdose. The five areas of PATHOS, on which the acronym is based, are:

- Have you ever had **P**roblems for longer than one month?
- Were you **A**lone at the time?
- Did you plan the overdose for longer than **T**hree hours?
- Are you feeling **HO**peless about the future?
- Were you feeling **S**ad for most of the time before the overdose?

The more features present, the greater the likelihood is of significant suicidal intent and depression. PATHOS has been used in emergency departments and can be helpful in determining hopelessness and intent surrounding further self-harm (Kingsbury 1993; Kingsbury 1996; Kumar *et al.* 2006).

FACE

Functional Analysis of the Care Environment (FACE) is a system and means of collecting information for the purpose of assessing individual needs and progress, measuring outcome and ensuring high-quality care. Including a focus on self-harm and suicide risk, the tools integrate the processes of assessment and outcomes measurement, and also include care planning and review documentation. The FACE Risk Assessment Package is a portfolio of risk assessment tools designed for a wide range of health and social care settings. It includes both screening and more detailed assessment, and includes specialist forms applicable to areas, such as mental health and young people.

STORM

The STORM Project for Children and Young Adults offers skills-based training in risk assessment and management of suicide and self-harm. It is aimed at frontline professionals in health, social and criminal justice services. Modules cover suicide and self-harm risk assessment, crisis management and prevention and self-help strategies. Packages are available separately or as part of a computer course.

Assessing self-harm and suicide in secure settings

We heard in an earlier chapter that young people in secure settings are at greater risk of self-harm than young people in general.

The ASSET tool is used across secure settings and is a screening instrument intended to capture basic needs, including those related to vulnerability and associated risks including self-harm. ASSET includes a pathway to specialist mental health assessment through SQUIFA (Screening Questionnaire Interview for Adolescents) and SIFA (Screening Interview for Adolescents), both mental health assessments for young people in secure settings. In particular, ASSET includes a Risk of Serious Harm Assessment; a Vulnerability Management Plan; and a Risk Management Plan.

In addition, the prison service uses the ACCT (Assessment, Care in Custody and Teamwork) system to respond to the vulnerable needs of young people in custody. The ACCT process sets out care planning and review objectives in relation to self-harm and suicide attempts. Collectively, these provide a mechanism to improve risk management related to suicide by young people in secure settings.

Young people who self-harm in secure settings may benefit from dialectical behaviour therapy (DBT), a treatment that has been used successfully with adult and young offenders in the UK and North America (McDougall and Jones 2007). Self-harm and suicide by young people in secure settings is increasingly recognised as a safeguarding issue (National Children's Bureau 2008; HM Treasury 2008).

What do we do with the risk assessment?

There is little point assessing risk without considering how best to address and manage the risk. The overall purpose of a risk assessment is to gain a broad understanding of why the young person is suicidal or self-harming, to explore what kind of help may be required and to encourage the young person to consider alternative, non-destructive coping strategies.

Health professionals and others must always be able to justify the decisions they make, regardless of whether the decisions are about meeting a young person's needs or managing their risk. This is particularly important when such decisions are likely to have safety and resource implications.

Risk can be both general and specific, and good management can reduce and prevent harm. Therefore, the management plan should involve developing one or more flexible strategies aimed at preventing the negative event from occurring or, if this is not possible, minimising the harm that may be caused.

Management plans

A comprehensive psychosocial risk assessment involves talking with the young person individually, meeting with their parents or carers and then making a collaborative management plan (Armstrong 2006). If, through the assessment process, it is established that the self-harm was not done with suicidal intent, then a plan needs to be made with the young person about the safest way to manage their self-harm. This should also include a plan of how to address the underlying problems, thus reducing the risks for further self-harm.

Factors that may trigger further episodes of self-harming or suicidal behaviour should always be recorded in a risk management plan, which is readily available to all those involved in the young person's care and treatment. It is important to actively involve the young person and their parents or carers in the development of the risk management plan, which should identify both chronic and acute risks. In addition, young people should be encouraged to identify alternatives to high-risk behaviours which may cause further harm.

Risk management plans must include clearly defined action points, where accountability for each aspect of the plan is allocated to a suitably qualified or experienced professional or other adult. All risk management plans should contain review dates.

Harm minimisation

In recent years, there has been a focus on harm minimisation in relation to self-harm and suicide. This focuses on the recognition that some people need to self-harm, and encourages their behaviours to remain within safe limits. Harm minimisation has mainly focused on self-injury, but has also included restricting access to the means of self-harm.

Applied inappropriately, harm minimisation strategies may give the message that self-harm by young people is to be encouraged rather than replaced. This concern becomes greater the younger a child is. This is not to say that the goal is to stop young people self-harming, rather that whilst they are exploring alternatives, guidance in relation to their self-harm focuses on safety and reducing the potential for long-term damage or death.

Is harm minimisation effective?

There has been a lack of research on the effects of restricting access to means of self-harm on rates of completed suicide (NHS Health Development Agency 2002). In addition, there has been little research investigating control of self-harm and suicide means.

For example, Hawton and colleagues (2009) explored the relationship between the use of lockable storage devices for pesticides and self-poisoning by people in Sri Lanka. Better controls in relation to easy access to pesticides by suicidal people had positive outcomes, and the researchers suggested that a larger scale trial was warranted.

Practical methods, such as reducing the availability of the means of self-harm can be helpful at both an individual and societal level (Cotgrove 2005). NICE recommends that for all children and young people, parents and carers should be advised to remove all means of self-harm, including medication, before the child or young person goes home from hospital (NICE 2004a).

Safety in overdose

The Department of Health's national suicide prevention strategy and reports identify the year following self-harm as a high-risk time for young people, and highlight the need to reduce access to significant quantities of medicines (Department of Health 2002b; Department of Health 2003). Many prescription medications have now been made safer in overdose. These include newer antidepressant drugs, such as selective serotonin reuptake inhibitors (SSRIs), which are less toxic in overdose than the older tricyclic antidepressants.

Safety warnings in general have been improved in product information, but some have argued that this may increase risk in some people for whom such information on overdose or poisoning may assist suicide. The various views about prescribing and self-poisoning in relation to UK regulatory authority warnings has had a significant effect on the use of SSRIs with young people under 18 (Bergen *et al.* 2009).

Whilst it is important to take an overall harm minimisation approach to self-harm, harm minimisation strategies should not be recommended for young people who ingest tablets and other poisons. This is because there are no safe limits in self-poisoning (NICE 2004a). Instead, advice about the toxic effects of poisoning should be given to the young person.

There is some evidence that restricting access to large quantities of over-the-counter medicines reduces the severity of adverse consequences of overdose. Children and young people who take overdoses often swallow para-cetamol (Clark *et al.* 2000; Hawton *et al.* 2001; Bhugra *et al.* 2004; Social Care Institute for Excellence 2005). This is partly because it is readily available in pharmacists, supermarkets and small shops and other outlets such as garages. Paracetamol is also available in combinations with other preparations, includ-ing decongestants and over-the-counter remedies, which increases the risk for accidental poisoning as well as self-harm (Farley *et al.* 2005).

When we consider that most self-harm by young people is impulsive, the availability of cheap, potentially lethal medication 24 hours a day should be cause for concern. Legislation passed in 1998 enforced blister packaging with reduced pack sizes of 16 tablets for over-the-counter sales of paracetamol. Due to the impulsive nature in which some overdoses are taken, blister packag-ing provides delays to help the person think about what they are doing. This makes the process of overdose slower, and packages generally contain fewer tablets than bottles. Findings strongly supporting this have been published since the legislation was passed, as results show a reduction in the amount of tablets taken in a single overdose (Hawton 2002; Turville *et al.* 2000).

Farley *et al.* (2005) go further, stating that a more direct health promo-tion message, involving the media, about the potentially fatal consequences of paracetamol poisoning may help reduce the number of impulsive self-harm attempts. This might be similar to the health promotion campaigns in the 1970s and 80s which helped to pass clear messages through generations of parents about keeping medicines and chemicals such as bleach, safely out of the reach of young children. Safety caps on bottles aided the goal of reducing accidental poisoning in this young age group.

Risk management and the Care Programme Approach

The Care Programme Approach (CPA) is the UK system of delivering hos-pital- and community-based mental health services. It was introduced in England in 1991 and by 1996 was in use across most specialist mental health services. Risk management is a key part of the CPA framework. The CPA involves identifying specific interventions based on an individual's support needs, taking into account safety and risk issues. Care plans should be drawn up to meet all of the service user's needs, including those needs relating to risk (Department of Health 2008).

Wider risk issues

The assessment of suicide risk involves an exploration of behaviour across several domains, including school, interpersonal relationships and social functioning. The presence of acute and chronic stress factors should be identified and recorded. Primary risk factors, including mood disorder, should be explored using direct questioning. This is to assess current ideation, intent and planning (Leighton 2006). Secondary risk factors, such as substance abuse and situational factors, such as family functioning, social support, and major life events all need to be explored using multiple methods and involving different people (Stanard 2000).

As we have seen, self-harm can be part of a complex picture, often accompanying other risky behaviours. It is therefore important to ensure that these other areas are also included in the assessment as well as the evaluation of self-harm and suicidal behaviour. Such behaviours include:

- aggression/violence/harm to others/property
- exposure to past/present physical/sexual/emotional abuse/domestic violence
- self-neglect
- exploitation.

Protective factors

When conducting an assessment as well as considering all the risk factors, protective factors also need to be considered. These are the aspects of a person's life that may help to reduce the impact of the risks they are facing. Protective factors can help facilitate positive outcomes, even when a young person is experiencing adverse life events and external stress. The following is a list of protective factors that support positive outcomes for young people who self-harm:

- Personal resources – emotional resilience
- Strong connections and supportive relationships with family and friends
- Evidence of ability to use problem solving skills and coping strategies
- Restricted access to lethal means of self-harm and suicide
- Access to supportive mental health, care or therapeutic relationship
- Enjoyment and involvement with school
- Life-affirming beliefs that discourage suicide and support self-preservation

Summary

A catalogue of child protection failures has resulted in organisations providing services for young people to become more risk averse. Sellen (2008) argues that the plethora of risk assessment and management tools and the pressure on frontline professionals and their managers to 'get it right' has created unhelpful anxiety within children's services.

All information which is gathered and corroborated during the assessment process is used to make judgements and decisions in relation to a young person's self-harm and risk of serious injury or death. This is based on a number of factors, including the young person's choice; issues of competence and capacity; the assessor's knowledge and experience; and the research evidence about what works for young people who self-harm. Rather than making decisions about risk in isolation, it is good practice to discuss risk assessments and management strategies with colleagues. This allows different perspectives to be considered and provides an opportunity to highlight issues that may have been overlooked.

Structured assessments can be helpful in assessing the risk of self-harm and suicide, but there are currently no instruments with a satisfactory evidence base. Therefore, a thorough and competent assessment should address precipitating factors, the context in which the self-harming or suicidal behaviour takes place and the role of psychosocial factors.

All tool-based risk assessments should be conducted as one part of a thorough and systematic overall clinical assessment. This is particularly important when assessing the risk of suicide and self-harm, as there is currently no instrument with a sufficiently strong evidence base or predictive power.

7 Treatments for young people who self-harm

Key points:

- The evidence base for the treatment of self-harm and suicidal behaviour by children and young people is extremely limited.
- Notwithstanding limitations in the knowledge base, available treatment options include individual psychological interventions, behavioural techniques, medication targeted at coexisting mental health problems, and both family therapy and group psychotherapy.
- Working in an honest and open way with young people and families is always the key to success. Sharing our views and generating and agreeing collaborative management plans is likely to enable positive outcomes. In contrast, unilateral decision making and paternalistic interventions are likely to be less successful.
- Individual therapy with young people who self-harm is often based on the principles of crisis intervention which is brief, intensive and focused on current difficulties.
- Although the number of studies is small, there is a relatively strong evidence base for group treatments on reducing the likelihood of self-harm repetition.
- Family-based interventions, whilst an important component of therapy or treatment, are rarely effective in isolation. Furthermore, family interventions are not suitable for all children and young people, particularly older adolescents.
- Multi-modal treatment strategies designed to support young people who self-harm should focus on social skills building, problem solving skills and care seeking behaviours.
- Treatment programmes for young people vary widely across the UK and include different forms of counselling, individual and group therapy and problem solving strategies, but there is currently not enough evidence to demonstrate which are the most effective.

Introduction

Working in an honest and open way with young people and families is always the key to success. Sharing our views and generating and agreeing collaborative management plans is likely to enable positive outcomes. By contrast, unilateral decision making and paternalistic interventions are likely to be less successful. Before any therapeutic work can take place with young people who self-harm, a trusting therapeutic relationship will need to be established in a climate of understanding and acceptance. This is part of the engagement process discussed in earlier chapters.

Promising treatments

The primary purpose of intervention with children and young people who are suicidal or self-harming is to prevent suicide, reduce repetition of self-harm and address the issues that combine to produce self-harm or suicidal behaviour. Secondary aims are to enhance psychological and social functioning and improve quality of life.

Treatment options include psychological interventions, behavioural techniques, medications targeted at coexisting mental health problems, family therapy and group psychotherapy. The mental state of the presenting young person can be complex and involve a host of environmental, interpersonal and internal difficulties. Although there are many different treatment strategies used, less evidence is available on whether these are effective or not.

Non-compliance with treatment is well documented, and Kreitman (1979) reported compliance in less than one-half of young people referred for deliberate self-harm. There are likely to be many reasons for this, but little is known about the effect of strategies to increase treatment compliance by children and young people who self-harm.

Individual therapies

Individual therapies generally aim to address the psychological factors that combine to cause and maintain self-harm or suicidal behaviour. These may include anxiety or depression, impulsivity or difficulties with problem solving. The principal aim of most individual psychological therapies is to enable people to adapt perspectives and develop alternative coping strategies and ways of expressing their feelings (Social Care Institute for Excellence 2005).

There are many different forms of individual therapy. Deciding which approach to use depends on the developmental status of the child, the evidence base for use and the specific wishes of the child, their family or carers. Expressive therapies, such as play or music therapy, may be appropriate for younger children, whereas older adolescents may benefit from talking therapies such as CBT or family therapy. Children with a low IQ or marked receptive speech difficulties and social impairment are less likely to benefit from talking therapies.

Creative therapies often have a psychodynamic basis and may be used on an individual or group basis. Some children may benefit more from using expressive or creative media, such as art, music or dance therapy (Nation 2003).

Individual therapy with young people who self-harm is often based, at least initially, on the principles of crisis intervention. Crisis or problem solving therapy is likely to be brief, intensive and focused on current difficulties. There is some evidence that problem solving therapy produces lower rates of repetition of self-harm during follow-up periods, although effect sizes are small (Department of Health 2003b).

Individual therapy varies considerably depending on the type of support needed by the particular young person. Most professionals tend to have their own framework of understanding the distress and a commitment to a particular kind of response. Such interventions range from counselling to more structured cognitive behavioural type strategies. Counsellors tend not to give advice or tell the young person how to solve their problems. Cognitive behavioural therapists are likely to be more directive and prescriptive about reaching resolution.

Cognitive therapies

Cognitive interventions are designed to change negative beliefs by gaining insight into how one's thoughts, feelings and behaviour are connected. Young people are helped to first elucidate, and then challenge, aspects of their core beliefs and negative thoughts (Woolley 2006). Cognitive behavioural therapy (CBT) is a discrete, time limited, structured psychological treatment. It is based on the premise that cognition is a primary determinant of behaviour and mood (Fonagy 2003).

Interventions are aimed at targeting and changing faulty cognitions to produce a change in affect and behaviour. Therefore, the removal of negatively distorted beliefs improves coping mechanisms. CBT interventions and problem solving strategies are used increasingly with young people who self-harm, and their use with adolescents has been shown to be effective (Wood *et al.* 1996; Harrington *et al.* 1998a; Rohde 2005). However, most of the studies that investigate outcomes and effectiveness involve teenagers and adults, and fewer studies have been conducted with younger adolescents and children.

There has been some evidence to suggest that cognitive behavioural therapies are effective in reducing suicidal behaviours (Salkovskis *et al.* 1990). Kolko and Brent (1988) demonstrated that 80 per cent of young people who engaged in a treatment programme of combined cognitive and interpersonal therapy showed remission for suicidal behaviour. Liberman and Eckman's (1981) study, highlighted earlier, compared a behaviour therapy approach with an insight orientated therapy with adults, and reported a relatively positive result with both groups. However, neither study included the additional treatments participants may have received, such as antidepressant medication.

Manual assisted cognitive therapy

Manual assisted cognitive therapy (MACT) was developed by Evans and colleagues as a brief, cognitively orientated and problem focused therapy comprising up to five sessions in three months of an episode of self-harm, with the option of a further two booster sessions within six months (Evans *et al.* 1999). There is evidence that MACT has some effect on reducing self-harm and suicidal acts in adults (Fagin 2006; Weinberg *et al.* 2006). However, there is a lack of research exploring MACT with young people under 18.

Problem solving therapy

Problem solving therapy is a brief psychological treatment for depression and is based on the principles of CBT (Huband *et al.* 2007). However, research with children and young people has been limited, and most studies have been conducted with adults. Problem solving techniques can be helpful in encouraging the young person to re-establish a sense of autonomy. Problem solving therapy as a brief psychological intervention has been used extensively as a form of crisis intervention following self-harm or attempted suicide (Hawton and Kirk 1989).

Through a collaborative process, the therapist forms a supportive relationship with the client whereby together they can clarify and work out which steps need to be taken to begin to solve the problems. In cognitive therapy, the therapist may assist the patient in recognising and re-appraising negative cognitions which threaten constructive action.

Like many individual therapy approaches, psychotherapeutic interventions aim to explore feelings, thoughts and experiences. The origins of current problems are viewed as being related to the past. Psychotherapy often involves more intensive, regular meetings and is likely to span a longer period of time. Role play, play therapy and other creative therapies may be used to enable the young person to use different mediums of communication.

Dialectical behaviour therapy

Dialectical behaviour therapy (DBT) is the only treatment known to be effective in reducing self-harm among people with borderline personality disorder. Earlier in the book, we mentioned that borderline personality and self-harm do not necessarily coexist, but for some people with borderline personality disorder, self-harm is a coping strategy. Various randomised controlled trials (RCTs) have shown that those who have had DBT have fewer suicidal ideas, are less likely to engage in self-harming behaviour and have fewer hospital admissions following self-harm (Koerner and Dimeff 2000; Dimeff *et al.* 2002).

The NICE guidelines on self-harm state that for people who self-harm and have a diagnosis of borderline personality disorder, consideration should be given to the use of DBT (NICE 2004a). DBT is also cited as an effective treatment in the NICE guidelines on the treatment and management of borderline personality disorder (National Collaborating Centre for Mental Health 2009).

What is DBT?

DBT is a cognitive behavioural psychotherapy based on biosocial theory pioneered by Marsha Linehan and colleagues at the Behavioural Research and Therapy Clinics in the USA. This was first used to treat the chronically para-suicidal behaviours of adult women. Although developed as an outpatient treatment, DBT has also been shown to be effective in other contexts, including inpatient units and forensic settings (Barley *et al.* 1993; Linehan *et al.* 1999; Bohus *et al.* 2001).

DBT is most commonly used to help people with borderline personality disorder manage their self-harm. This is achieved by developing self-awareness, reducing impulsivity and through emotional regulation and positive coping strategies. DBT comprises a programme of individual and group therapy, social skills training and access to crisis management by telephone. DBT has been adapted to use with young people, particularly those who repeatedly self-harm (Miller *et al.* 2007).

Linehan describes the features of borderline personality disorder in terms of 'dysregulation'. This means that people often struggle with their sense of self and frequently describe feeling empty, unreal or 'cut off'. Therapists at the Behavioural Research and Therapy Clinics refer to dysregulation in cognitive, affective, behavioural and interpersonal terms (see Table 7.1). People with borderline personality disorder are emotionally vulnerable. They may have unrealistic goals and expectations, feeling angry or worthless if they struggle or fail to achieve these.

Due to extreme emotional reactions, people with borderline personality disorder frequently have a chaotic lifestyle. In an attempt to cope with intolerable feelings of stress they may engage in suicidal, self-harming or impulsive behaviours. DBT aims to help people with borderline personality disorder to decrease destructive, self-harming or life-threatening behaviours, and improve their overall quality of life.

DBT is based on a biosocial theory which suggests that borderline personality disorder evolves as a consequence of an emotionally vulnerable person growing up within an 'invalidating environment' (Linehan 1993a). Linehan defines an emotionally vulnerable person as one whose autonomic nervous system reacts excessively to stress, and is slow to return to a normal baseline. An invalidating environment is a situation where a child's emotional responses are ignored by significant others such as their parents.

As the name suggests, DBT places emphasis on dialectics and there is no absolute truth. Young people are encouraged to recognise that reality is complex, and that contradictory thoughts and views are both inevitable and can be synthesised. In DBT, the relationship between client and therapist

Table 7.1 DSM-IV criteria for borderline personality disorder

Affective dysregulation	Unstable mood; which may be episodic, intense and associated with anxiety or irritability. This usually lasts a few hours, and rarely more than several days
	Anger which may be intense, inappropriate or poorly controlled. This may manifest as temper tantrums, displays of anger and physical fights
Behavioural dysregulation	Potentially self-destructive impulsivity in at least two areas of functioning. This may include sexual behaviour, substance abuse or binge eating. Suicidal or self-mutilating behaviour is not included. Recurrent suicidal gestures or threats of self-mutilating behaviour are included
Interpersonal dysregulation	Efforts to avoid abandonment which may be real or imagined
	Unstable and intense interpersonal relationships characterised by extremes of devaluation and idealisation
Self dysregulation	Disturbance of self identity and self image, and chronic feelings of emptiness
Cognitive dysregulation	Brief, stress related paranoid ideas or extreme dissociative symptoms

is considered to be highly influential in the success of treatment. The most fundamental dialectic of all involves accepting the young person as they are. This is in the context of supporting them to change, to be comfortable with change, and to develop non-destructive coping strategies.

Dialectic strategies used in DBT enable the young person and therapist to balance change and acceptance, and reduce the potential for both people getting stuck with rigid thoughts and behaviours. Therapists receive supervision as part of therapists' consultation groups. This is intended to enhance therapeutic capabilities and prevent burnout.

The four stages of DBT

Young people with emerging borderline personality disorder often have multiple interpersonal problems and struggle with coping with stress and conflict. Deciding where to start is often difficult for both the young person and therapist. For this reason, agreeing what to focus on and when is one of the first tasks in DBT. This is addressed through a four-stage treatment hierarchy (see Table 7.2). The pre-treatment stage focuses on assessment, commitment and orientation. This is to assess motivation to change and set achievable goals.

Table 7.2 Four-stage DBT treatment hierarchy

Therapy stage	Focuses on
Pre treatment	Assessment, commitment and orientation
1	Suicidal behaviours, therapy interfering behaviours and behaviours that interfere with quality of life
2	Post-traumatic stress
3	Self-esteem and individual treatment goals

Stage 1 focuses on suicidal behaviours, therapy interfering behaviours, and behaviours which interfere with quality of life. Stage 2 deals with post-traumatic stress. Stage 3 focuses on self-esteem and individual treatment goals. The targeted behaviours that are being addressed at one stage are brought under control before moving on to the next stage. This is achieved using a range of therapeutic strategies which include validation and problem solving.

Individual therapy

In DBT, the relationship between the young person and therapist is thought to be highly influential in the success of therapy. DBT is a collaborative therapy and requires a lot of motivation from both the young person and their therapist. Weekly therapy sessions are provided, structured around the young person's diary card. This is used to monitor target behaviours, the intensity of emotions they experience, and the new skills that are being learned (see Table 7.3).

If a young person harms themself between individual sessions they are expected to complete a 'chain analysis'. This involves a detailed behavioural analysis of the events that led to the self-harm, and can help identify likely reinforcing contingencies for the maladaptive behaviours that followed. Between sessions, young people are offered telephone support from their individual therapist. The focus of this is to support young people in their application of adaptive skills learned during individual therapy sessions.

Skills training group

Young people receiving DBT also attend a skills training programme comprising four modules. These are used to help the young person modulate their emotions and behaviours (see Table 7.4). Although the module on 'mindfulness' is always completed first, subsequent modules on interpersonal effectiveness, emotional regulation and distress tolerance can be completed in any order. The final module called 'Walking the Middle Path' is specifically for adolescents.

Table 7.3 Example of young person's diary card

DIARY CARD

Name: ....

Week commencing: ....

		Day						
		Mon	Tues	Wed	Thur	Fri	Sat	Sun
Urges								
Self-harm	0–5							
Suicide	0–5							
Other	0–5							
Emotions								
Pain	0–5							
Sad	0–5							
Shame	0–5							
Anger	0–5							
Fear	0–5							
Other	0–5							
Actions								
Self-harm	0–5							
Other	0–5							
*Skills	0–7							

*Urges
    0   no urges
    5   extremely strong urges

*Skills used

0	not thought about
1	thought about, not used, didn't want to
2	thought about, not used, wanted to
3	tried but couldn't use them
4	tried, could use them, but didn't help
5	tried, could use them, helped
6	didn't try, used them, didn't help
7	didn't try, used them, helped

Table 7.4 DBT skills training group

Module 1	Mindfulness
Module 2	Interpersonal effectiveness
Module 3	Emotion regulation
Module 4	Distress tolerance
Module 5	Walking the middle path (adolescents)

The concept of 'mindfulness' is at the centre of DBT. This refers to the ability to be in control of your own mind instead of letting your mind be in control of you (Linehan 1993b). Young people learn the difference between what Linehan calls the reasonable, emotional and wise mind. The reasonable mind is portrayed as logical, rational and focused and thoughts are 'cool'. In contrast, an emotional mind is controlled by current feelings. 'Hot' thoughts drive emotions, logical thinking becomes difficult and reality is distorted. The wise mind integrates the reasonable and emotional mind, and adds intuitive knowing so that the wise mind knows something to be true or valid. As part of mindfulness, young people are supported to focus on the present moment, rather than past or future events.

The second module focuses on interpersonal effectiveness training. This enables young people to deal with situations of conflict and develop self-respect. They are taught how to make their wants and needs known to others, respectfully and assertively, and how to say no to unreasonable requests or demands.

In the third module, young people are supported to develop skills to regulate their emotional responses. This involves recognising, labelling and managing strong emotions, such as sadness and anger. Young people learn that complete emotional control cannot be achieved, and that being emotional is a normal part of life.

The fourth skills training module focuses on distress tolerance. There is often a connection between an inability to tolerate strong emotions and impulsive behaviour which can serve to reduce intolerable distress. During this module, young people work on skills to manage anxiety or upset without making impulsive decisions, including self-harm.

Walking the middle path

DBT has been adapted for use with adolescents (DBT-A). This is with the primary focus of supporting young people and their families cope with the transition from adolescence to adulthood and manage the stresses and strains of family-based interpersonal relationships. A fifth skills module has been developed to teach adolescents and their parents about the concepts of dialectics, validation and reinforcement.

Multi-family skills training

Recognising that young people who self-harm often live with parents and carers, Alex Miller and colleagues have developed a DBT multi-family skills training group for adolescents and their parents or guardians (Miller *et al.* 2007). The 24-week skills-training programme includes weekly homework and the generalisation of new skills to real-life situations.

Multi-systemic therapy

Multi-systemic therapy (MST) is an evidence-based treatment from the USA. It is an intensive, home and family-based treatment combining family and cognitive behavioural strategies with a range of other family support services. A typical MST intervention lasts between four and six months and the service is on call 24 hours a day, seven days a week. Each MST therapist has a caseload of three to five young people and is expected to adapt their working pattern so they are available at times convenient to their service users or to respond to a crisis.

MST has been shown to reduce attempted suicide among children and adolescents. Young people presenting in psychiatric crisis were randomly assigned to MST or hospitalisation (Huey *et al.* 2004). Indices of attempted suicide, suicidal ideation, depressive affect and parental control were assessed before treatment, at four months after recruitment and at one year post-treatment follow-up. MST was found to be significantly more effective than emergency hospitalisation at reducing rates of attempted suicide, and symptom reduction over time was better for young people receiving MST. However, since the study group included psychotic and aggressive young people as well as those who were suicidal or self-harming, the population was not entirely consistent with the outcome being examined (Social Care Institute for Excellence 2005).

Family therapy

Since children grow up in families or alternative families, many solutions to problems can be found in the family context. Family therapy is based on the principles of a systemic or contextual approach (Woolley 2006). Although the two most common are strategic family therapy and structural family therapy, other techniques including narrative, psycho-educational, behavioural and Milan family therapy are also used. Techniques used in strategic family therapy include challenging rigid or absent boundaries, unbalancing the family equilibrium by temporarily joining with one family member against others, and setting 'homework' tasks designed to restore hierarchies (Asen 2002).

Randomised controlled trials have not shown family therapy to be as effective as other interventions for young people who self-harm (Senior 2003). However, since family dysfunction and poor relationships are predictors of persistence, it is common sense that family intervention alongside other treatments is likely to be helpful. There is some evidence that family dysfunction and poor communication between family members is associated with self-harm (Kerfoot *et al.* 1995; Kerfoot *et al.* 1996; Harrington 2001; Chitsabesan *et al.* 2003).

Much of the literature on the treatment of suicidal young people also suggests that family therapy or family involvement is an important component in treatment. There have been frequent reports on family dysfunction and on the family's lack of understanding and knowledge about suicidal behaviour. Some theorists have advocated a didactic intervention where parents receive a psycho-educational approach to help them understand the young person's dilemma.

Harrington *et al.* (1998b) used a brief home-based family intervention which targeted difficulties, such as poor communication and difficulties with problem solving. Family therapists may work with one whole family or a particular subgroup, for example mother and daughter. In many cases however, the family may not be motivated or compliant with treatment, making the role of family work even more complex. Kolko and Brent (1988) noted the importance of combining individual psychotherapies and family systemic approaches in the treatment of suicidal young people.

A team in Leeds are currently planning to conduct the SHIFT (Self-Harm Intervention Family Therapy) trial – a large multi-centred trial of a manualised family therapy 12-week programme. This aims to prevent self-harm repetition, and is discussed further in Chapter 10. While much has been reported about strong associations with family dysfunction and self-harm, family therapy is rarely effective as the sole treatment, nor is it recommended for all suicidal youngsters, particularly older adolescents.

Brief solution focused therapy

Brief solution focused therapy (BSFT) is aimed at building solutions rather than solving problems (Iverson 2002). A small number of studies have demonstrated positive outcomes with children and young people (Zimmerman *et al.* 1996; Lethem 1994; Rhodes and Ajmal 2004). BSFT aims to produce change and to enable the young person to recognise why change has occurred.

Using a scale between one and ten, Iverson (2002) suggests that improvement can be tracked, and explanations for what has caused such improvements can be identified. Comparing the different ratings provided by young people and their parents or carers can be helpful in understanding family relationships, perceptions of difficulties and coping styles within the family.

Group treatment

Group therapy is based on the premise that children's difficulties develop within a network of relationships and in the social context. Relationships are explored as part of a dynamic and changing process. Children and young people are able to discuss problems, identify with others and share strategies to resolve conflict and distress (Woolley 2006).

Group therapy has been used to treat a wide range of difficulties experienced by young people (Scheidinger and Aronson 1991). However, it has been seldom used with adolescents who self-harm. A group therapy programme for adolescents who repeatedly self-harmed found that group therapy was more effective at reducing future instances of self-harm than routine care (Wood *et al.* 2001). Most treatments to date have focused on individual therapy. This may be partly due to anxieties about grouping suicidal people together in case of issues of contagion or imitation of self-harm. In addition, there has been a lack of training for therapists in this modality.

Although psychotherapists sometimes recommend that suicidal people should be excluded from groups there has been no evidence to suggest that group therapy can be detrimental or harmful. Young people tend to want to belong to groups, and there is evidence from practice that suggests young people who self-harm identify with each other and often form covert groups. Through the evolution of social networking sites and other internet based resources, virtual groups of self-harmers have been developing. However, their impact on rates of self-harm and suicide is not known (WHO 2000a; Whitlock *et al.* 2006).

Feedback from young people suggests that they tend to find group treatment more attractive, and young people describe many positives, particularly reducing their sense of isolation and the promotion of social inclusion. Again, like many therapies, group therapies can be used in conjunction with other treatments. The NICE guidelines on self-harm (NICE 2004a) suggest that developmental group psychotherapy could be offered to young people. Similarly, group dialectical behavioural therapy has shown promise for suicidal adolescents in the USA (Miller *et al.* 2007). Both treatments involve the group programme being added to other approaches.

Psychopharmacological interventions

Psychotropic drugs can be used in the treatment of self-harm particularly when there is evidence of co-morbidity, such as anxiety states, psychosis and depressive symptomatology. However, treating children and young people with psychoactive medication is controversial. Use of medication with suicidal young people needs to be a cautious undertaking, given the high level of toxicity and fatal consequences of some drugs in overdose. Rettersol (1993) reported an increase in antidepressant overdose as a method for suicide. Reynolds and Mazza (1993), on the other hand, demonstrated efficacy in reducing suicidal ideations with antidepressants in the adult population.

Selective serotonin reuptake inhibitors (SSRIs), such as fluoxetine, are often the drug of choice for adolescents because they have fewer side effects and are safer in overdose. However, a systematic review by Whittington *et al.* (2004) reported that, with the exception of fluoxetine, SSRIs offer more risks than benefits to children and young people. The NICE guidelines on depression in children and young people recommends that those prescribed an antidepressant should be closely monitored for the appearance of suicidal behaviour, self-harm or hostility (National Collaborating Centre for Mental Health 2005).

Although some evidence supporting the use of depot flupenthixol has emerged from a systematic review on interventions for repeated self-harm in adults (Hawton *et al.* 1998b), there is no evidence to support its use with young people. Since injecting young people with slow-release antipsychotic medication is arguably even more controversial than using oral antidepressants, these drugs have rarely been considered as a frontline treatment for self-harm in young people unless, of course, self-harm co-occurs with psychosis (Pryjmachuk and Trainor in press).

A recent randomised controlled trial conducted in Manchester and Cambridge (Goodyer *et al.* 2007) found no benefit for CBT combined with an SSRI antidepressant over the use of an SSRI alone. This study provoked an ongoing debate among clinicians and researchers, and focused debate on the use of antidepressant medication and psychological treatments for children and adolescents (Cotgrove 2007; Timimi 2007).

Complimentary therapies

There is a lack of evidence about the impact of complimentary therapies on self-harm and suicidal behaviour. People often report that massage, meditation, aromatherapy and homeopathy can alleviate stress, and creative therapies such as those which use art, music or dance may be helpful in enabling expression, articulating thoughts and feelings and channelling distress (SANE 2007).

Conclusions

The evaluation and treatment of adolescent self-harm and suicide is an under-researched area of work in both the UK and the USA. A number of studies have been conducted to investigate epidemiological factors and risk indicators, but there is little robust evidence about treatments that are known to be effective.

Some of the promising individual treatments have been highlighted in this chapter. Although there has been a significant increase in interventions over the past ten years, there is currently no standard treatment in the UK or USA that is seen to be more superior than another. However, what seems clear is that high quality longitudinal studies are required with young people who self-harm and those at risk of suicide. Time and money can be wasted, and opportunities lost, by providing interventions that are not evidence-based nor produce good outcomes for children and young people.

8 Involving parents and carers

Key points:

- Numerous reports have highlighted that parental involvement is often woefully inadequate, and on occasions parents are excluded from professional care and treatment decisions at the most basic of levels.
- If a child or young person does not wish their parent or carer to be involved, every effort should be made to fully understand the reasons for this. This is not to apply pressure, but is to enquire if any steps could be taken to address the reasons why a young person may not want their parent or carer involved.
- Seeing, or being aware of, one's child hurting themselves and putting their life at risk can be very distressing for those around them. It is therefore important to address the impact of self-harm on parents, carers and other family members.
- The natural reaction for parents or carers is often to want to protect and take control of the situation. However, this may sometimes be counterproductive and they may sometimes need to be supported to get the balance right.
- Feeling helpless can influence parental behaviour and parenting interventions, leaving people feeling paralysed. Many describe a sense of 'walking on egg shells' or being 'held at ransom', and are wary of setting limits and boundaries. This leaves parents feeling disempowered, anxious and worried. These anxieties can be exacerbated by a lack of information and support from some health professionals.
- When parents or carers have been directly involved in the care and treatment of their son or daughter it is important to ask about their experience of this. This is so the service can reflect on whether parents and carers feel listened to, that their views are being considered and that they have been appropriately involved.

Introduction

Depending on the different organisational or community context in which adults come into contact with young people who self-harm, the degree and extent to which parents and carers may be involved will vary. However, it is essential to remember what to some may at first seem obvious – the majority of children and young people have parents or carers and many will want them to be involved to some degree.

This chapter explores some examples of how parents or carers can be appropriately involved when their son or daughter is suicidal or self-harming. It addresses some of the key issues that need to be considered, as well as discusses some of the more complex issues that may arise.

Policy context

Parents and carers' involvement in care and treatment decisions is at the heart of the modernisation of the NHS and its component structures, organisations and services. The National Service Framework for Children, Young People and Maternity Services includes a detailed standard on supporting parents and carers (Department of Health 2004). This sets out the requirements of services to work together so that parents and carers are properly involved, have access to appropriate information and have the support they need in looking after and meeting the needs of their children.

The Health Advisory Service points out that parents of teenagers are often the last group to be seen as a resource, and yet they are, more often than any other group of adults, the first person a child or young person confides in (Health Advisory Service 1994). In recent years, the profile of 'involvement' has been raised and NHS organisations have developed strategies for public and patient involvement (PPI). This takes many forms, including the employment of service users and carers who contribute to the planning, delivery and evaluation of the organisation's activities.

What do we mean by parental involvement?

It is important to discuss what we mean by involving parents and carers. Whereas most children and young people live with a family member, some are looked after by the local authority. In this chapter, the term carer is used to refer to an adult with responsibility for a child or young person. This may involve parental responsibility or a more general responsibility for a child's welfare or well-being. Of course, many children and young people have parents as well as carers. This includes those who have residential respite care or who are living away from home in hospital. Such care is provided by an adult in a *loco parentis* role.

It is important to be clear that involvement per se is not a specific activity. Rather, it is a process and refers to a range of different interventions which vary in frequency and intensity according to the issue being considered.

Why is involving parents important?

Whilst it is important to be clear about consent and confidentiality, it is essential that professionals and other adults take every opportunity to appropriately involve parents wherever their child or young person may be living or receiving a service. This is because the majority of children and young people live with one or both parents, and involving them in their care in some way is a matter of common sense. In addition, in a large scale survey of young people's life experiences, support from family was identified as being key to overall well-being (Princes Trust 2009).

Research into child heath and well-being suggests that British youngsters have among the worst relationships with parents in Europe (UNICEF 2007). In a study of 100 young people admitted to hospital following an episode of self-harm, 47 per cent identified a serious disagreement with a parent during the previous 24 hours as the main reason for their self-harm (Kerfoot 1988). This suggests that the relationship a young person has with their parents or carers may be directly connected to their suicidal or self-harming behaviour. Therefore, parental involvement is likely to be necessary in understanding and addressing the difficulties involved.

Chapter 5 highlighted the importance of collecting information from a range of different sources. This is to assist the professional in formulating their understanding about what a young person's suicidal or self-harming behaviour is about. Parents and carers usually know their children much better than professionals, and often have views about what their son or daughter's, self-harm or suicidal behaviour is about. Parents can also provide a developmental history, sometimes crucial in determining when a young person's difficulties began, and how they have evolved. Notwithstanding issues of confidentiality, it is therefore important to seek their views.

How can we properly involve parents and carers?

Despite the obvious principles which have been discussed so far, numerous reports have highlighted that parental involvement is often woefully inadequate. All too often, parents are excluded from professional care and treatment decisions at the most basic of levels. This is despite clear messages in research and policy documents that parental involvement is of central importance.

Some organisations have attempted to address this situation by publishing strategies to involve and support parents at every level of service planning and delivery. *Parent Power* is Tameside's parent plan which aims to empower parents of vulnerable children, including those who are suicidal or self-harming. Recognising that some parents require additional support, the strategy has key priorities, including emotional health and well-being.

Thameside's Power, *Parent Power* Strategy and action plan

1   All service plans for children and young people and their families should indicate how they will include and support parents.
2   Services will recognise their role in supporting parents by mapping their position on the Parenting Support Framework to reflect the different levels of support that parents require.
3   Parent support will be developed and delivered to meet the needs of parents.
4   Parents know about what is available.
5   Develop a local delivery model for parenting courses and informal support.
6   Develop a skilled and knowledgeable workforce to provide quality parent support.
7   Parents have the opportunity to influence services for children and young people.
8   Parent support and involvement is adequately funded.
9   Parent support and involvement is monitored and evaluated.

(Thameside Children and Young People
Strategic Partnership 2008)

Achieving a balance

People who self-harm should be allowed, if they wish, to be accompanied by a family member, friend or advocate during the assessment or treatment process (NICE 2004a). Indeed, many children and young people want their parents to be present, particularly during initial assessments. However, young people should always be offered the opportunity to speak alone. This is in order to maintain confidentiality and allow discussion about issues and problems that are directly associated with family members and relationships.

> Time on your own is important as there are some things you wouldn't want to say in front of your parents. You can be worried to say certain things as it can cause arguments when you get home.
>
> Lauren, 17

Some services are designed and organised in a way that includes parents directly in the assessment and treatment or therapy process. For example, in specialist CAMHS, parents are usually present for at least some of initial assessments, and in some cases subsequent treatment sessions. Whilst the young person may be having individual sessions or group work, there may be sessions arranged for the parents on their own, or the work may involve family therapy, seeing part of or the whole family together.

It is always important to sensitively explore views about information sharing. If a child or young person does not wish their parent or carer to be involved in decisions about their self-harm, every effort should be made to fully understand the reasons for this. This is not to apply pressure on the child or young person to share information they do not wish to share, but to enquire if any steps could be taken to address the reasons why a young person may not want their parent or carer involved. This requires a careful balance of enquiry and respect for privacy, and young people should never be made to feel pressured about decisions involving parents and carers.

When parents refuse to be involved

It is not always young people who decide they do not want their parents to be involved. Sometimes, parents choose not to be involved themselves and refuse to cooperate with the young person's or professional's request to contribute to the assessment or therapy process. Perhaps not surprisingly, research has shown that young people who have uncooperative parents are more likely to repeat their self-harm. Refusing to allow the young person home following treatment in hospital for self-harm, or refusal to remove medicines from easy access are both risk factors for further self-harm. Sometimes, this may be a parent's initial reaction as they are finding it hard to deal with their own feelings and put the needs of their child first. At other times these uncooperative behaviours represent a serious breakdown in parenting, and in some circumstances social services need to be informed and may become involved.

The paediatrician and child psychoanalyst Donald Winnicott coined the term a 'good enough mother' to refer to someone who provides unconditional love, care and consistency for their child. This includes physical and emotional nurture and protection such as warmth and praise, in order for their child to grow into a healthy, secure adult. The 'good enough' parent is in contrast to the unrealistic and unhelpful notion of a 'perfect mother' (Winnicott 1965). The vast majority of parents are considered 'good enough' parents and manage to meet their child's needs. However, some struggle, and perhaps have not received what they would consider as good enough parenting. They may have an idea they want to be different, but putting these ideas consistently into action can be difficult.

Sharing difficult situations

Parents often share the same worries as the young person. For example, they may have been concerned about their low mood for some time, or worry that friendships are becoming strained. Together, they may have thought about getting help or may have already approached services for help. At other times, parents may be completely unaware of their child's self-harm or not know that they were feeling suicidal. They may express surprise or be dismayed that all had seemed normal. Oldershaw (2008) describes how parents and young people sometimes share ambivalence about seeking help, together hoping that problems will resolve themselves.

It is important to put the account given by the young person and the parents or carers together. This is to help make sense of both the episode of self-harm and the underlying factors. When parental accounts of self-harm are very similar to young people's, it can indicate that they are in touch with each other and share a close, caring relationship. However, this is often not the case, and accounts may differ considerably. The young person may have been showing their distress for some time but the parent may not have noticed. It is not unusual for young people to have been keeping their distress and self-harm well hidden. Indeed, by all accounts the self-harm may have come 'out of the blue' and not occur in the context of other problems that parents may be aware of.

Young people can often be supported to involve their parents in understanding and addressing their self-harming behaviour. This does not need to be an all-or-nothing situation. They may agree to share the main themes, such as warning signs that they are struggling, or strategies to help keep them safe, but make some exceptions to information sharing. For example, they may consider that things they wish to remain private have little or no bearing on the current situation. For example, they may smoke cigarettes or be engaged in a sexual relationship and request that this information is kept confidential.

Sometimes young people agree that their parents should know about self-harm, but not want them to know how long this has been happening. Other times they may only agree to minimal involvement, which might include knowing that their son or daughter is attending therapy sessions to talk to someone. Occasionally, young people refuse to have parents involved at all, even to be informed that they are having, or are in need of, help.

How parents might be feeling

It is important to address the impact of self-harm on parents, carers and other family members. Seeing or being aware of one's child hurting themselves and putting their life at risk can be very distressing for those around them. The NICE guidelines on self-harm advise that professionals should provide emotional support and help if necessary to the relatives or carers of people who have self-harmed (NICE 2004a).

As well as gaining additional information to help build a bigger picture of the self-harm or suicidal behaviour, it is important to give parents an opportunity to express how they feel and explore how this may impact on the recovery of the young person. Anger, self-blame and helplessness have each been reported as parental responses to self-harm by their son or daughter (Raphael *et al.* 2006).

Parental perspectives on their child's self-harm have not been widely published. One study concluded that parents often spot signs of self-harm early on, but need more help and support in how to deal with it (Oldershaw 2008).

Byrne *et al.* (2008) conducted a study to identify the support needs of parents and carers of young people who had self-harmed. Focus groups highlighted the following themes as important:

- support
- information about self-harm
- skills for parenting
- managing future incidents
- communication
- relationships
- discipline.

An eight-week parenting group called SPACE was developed from the study which aimed to address these key themes (Byrne *et al.* 2008).

Another study that recruited parents of young people attending CAMHS for support with repetitive self-harm showed that parents experienced feelings of shock, disappointment, guilt, fear, sadness and a sense of loss (Oldershaw *et al.* 2008). The researchers found that parents benefited from advice and support, either individually or in a group, to help them manage their child's self-harming behaviour. They noted that even those with prior knowledge of self-harm and an intellectual understanding of the issues struggled to come to terms with and manage these behaviours by their own child.

This ambivalence needs to be discussed, along with other parental feelings, so as to help and support the parent and influence the young person in the most helpful way. For example, non-attendance at appointments may be as much to do with parental ambivalence as uncertainty on the part of the child or young person themself.

Shock and distress

Listening to someone who is distressed, even for professionals, can be extremely demanding and upsetting, and this is why there are professional systems such as clinical supervision. There is no doubt that self-harm or suicidal behaviour by a son or daughter can be an extremely traumatic experience for parents. Parents are often devastated when their child self-harms, either by overdose or through self-injury, such as cutting or burning. Their natural reaction is often to want to protect and take control of the situation. However, this may sometimes be counterproductive.

> I can't believe my daughter would do this, the thought of her cutting herself makes me want to cry. I have brought her up to protect her from harm and now this is happening.
>
> Angie

As difficult as it may be, it is important for parents or carers to be as understanding and supportive as possible about their child's self-harm. This is no easy task and some parents simply cannot cope with seeing someone they love harm themselves. The relationship a parent has with their child is different to the one that a professional has with a child, and parents often need to be supported to remain calm and manage their own feelings of upset and distress. This is if they are to be helpful and not make things worse.

Helplessness

Parents often report feeling powerless, helpless and out of control when their child self-harms. In a study by Raphael (2006), parents expressed concerns about coping with their child on discharge from hospital, and were worried about the possibility of future incidents. Some parents struggle with putting their child's needs ahead of their own. The self-harming behaviour of their son or daughter may resonate with the past experiences of parents and generate strong negative feelings. For example, past experiences of bullying or abuse may reawaken feelings of helplessness, disempowerment and loss of control in the parent or carer.

Parents have learnt a lot about how to be a parent from their own experiences of childhood and being parented. Some parents find it helpful to reflect on the ways in which they themselves were parented. This allows them to consider alternatives, make adjustments and reconsider or revise parenting strategies. It is important for parents to recognise their own issues and set these aside from those which belong to their son or daughter. Being aware of these processes means parents can address them, and often, the awareness that they are different people in different circumstances is sufficient.

Feeling helpless can influence parental behaviour and parenting interventions and leave people feeling paralysed. Many describe a sense of 'walking on egg shells' or being 'held at ransom', and are wary of setting limits and boundaries. This leaves them disempowered, anxious and worried. These anxieties can be exacerbated by a lack of information and support from some health professionals. However setting appropriate rules and providing consistent boundaries that produce a sense of safety, security and containment is an important part of a parent's role with a young person who is suicidal or self-harming. However, for some parents or carers, this is not as easy as it sounds, and professional support may be required.

Exclusion

Some young people do not want their parents to be involved, and others want only minimal involvement. Whilst informed decisions by young people need to be respected, this can leave parents feeling excluded and wondering what is troubling their son or daughter. As we discussed earlier, the transition from childhood to adulthood sees a move from dependence to independence, with increased importance placed on the peer group rather than parents or carers. This can often include the blanket exclusion of parents in all things personal and private.

We have also heard that many young people remain ambivalent about parental involvement, and some need to be reassured that their parents are available, even though they may be reluctant to admit it. Therefore, the involvement of parents and carers should be seen as an evolutionary process. Again, this is not to cajole young people into sharing information they do not wish to divulge, but it is about recognising that adolescence is a period of transition and young people often change their minds.

Parents can be reassured by hearing that their experiences of struggling to support their son or daughter are not unusual. It can be validating to hear that being ignored for hours on end or being the repository for all the problems in the world is part of parenting an adolescent. It is not unusual for teenagers to spend hours alone in their rooms or immersed in the cyber world, or to use the house like a hotel, coming in to eat and expecting to be waited on hand and foot. Quite understandably, parents of young people who self-harm often struggle with this. Evidently it is still their job to look after their child physically, but faced with self-harm which is usually a sign of distress, they are excluded emotionally.

Young people are not expert problem solvers. They are still experimenting with problem solving and relationship management and will get things wrong some of the time. Unlike adults, they do not have the benefit of extensive life experience on their side, and this is where parents can be supportive. Parents are often reassured to hear that exclusion may be perfectly normal.

Kerry's choice

Kerry, aged 15, took an overdose of ten paracetamol tablets following pressure of exams and an argument with her boyfriend. She called for an ambulance herself and was admitted to hospital. Kerry's parents were away for the weekend and she was at home with her 19-year-old brother.

None of her family know about the overdose and Kerry is adamant she does not want them to know. She is medically fit for discharge.

The professional and Kerry discuss the reasons why Kerry does not want her parents to know about her overdose and why the professional thinks her parents should know – Kerry lives with her parents, they care for her, they help her sort out issues at school with her exams and have supported her during a split from her boyfriend.

Kerry says she feels stupid and that she has broken her parents trust. She says the overdose was impulsive. She reports that she has never done anything like this before and is adamant that she will not harm herself again. She wants no one to know and now just wants to get on with her life.

Putting all factors together the outcome of the risk assessment suggests that Kerry is at low risk of further self-harm or suicide.

In situations such as Kerry's, professionals should always try to involve parents in the care of their daughter or son as this is recognised as best practice in engaging young people and families or carers. Whilst the dilemma surrounding Kerry's choice does occur, in most cases young people who self-harm can be persuaded to recognise the importance of support from a responsible adult and agree that their parents should be involved.

However, when a young person refuses to have parents involved, professionals need to:

a) Assess whether the child or young person is competent or has capacity. This is discussed further in chapter 11.

b) Complete an individual risk and needs assessment, which may indicate low, medium, or high risk of further self-harm, and subsequently develop a robust management plan. This is discussed further in chapters 5 and 6.

c) Consider the welfare of the child or young person. Where there are concerns about safety and the young person is considered to be at risk of significant harm then confidentiality can be breached whether the young person is competent or not.

There are often no straightforward solutions to such dilemmas. It is important for professionals to balance the young person's right to confidentiality with the principle of parental involvement in the health and welfare of their child. This is in the context of the safety and welfare of the child. Whilst many parents have knowledge of the law and can appreciate their child's rights, it is understandable when some find this situation difficult and believe they have a right to know what is happening to their son or daughter. These issues are discussed further in chapter 11.

Involving parents in risk management

Discussions and decisions about parental involvement should always take place in the context of a therapeutic relationship between the young person and the professional. This provides a framework of trust, honesty and respect where collaboration and agreement can often be reached.

However, there are exceptions to the degree of collaboration, limits to confidentiality and circumstances in which the young person's right to confidentiality may be overruled. This is where the risks of not sharing information are considered too high, and maintaining confidentiality may lead to significant harm. The welfare of the child is paramount, and the limits to confidentiality need to be made explicit to the young person.

In practice, this means that if a person is self-harming safely and is unlikely to cause themselves any significant harm, their confidentiality need not be breached. In contrast, there are circumstances in which a young person who is actively suicidal may have their rights to confidentiality overruled, and informing others, including their parents or carers is necessary as part of a risk management plan.

When a young person has definite plans to achieve death by suicide, involvement of their parents or carers is crucial. This is to minimise the risks, keep the young person safe and, where possible, address the underlying issues to help reduce suicidal feelings. Parents' views about this, as well as those of the young person and the professionals, are central. A written management plan needs to be implemented, and where the risks are considered too high to manage in the community, the plan may involve inpatient hospital admission.

Helping to keep the young person safe

Parents have a key role to play in keeping a child or young person safe. The greater the concern about risk and safety, the more likely it is that parents will need to be fully involved. The management plan following self-harm has safety as its overall objective. Parents need to be involved in reducing the risk of further self-harm and this will involve recognising signs of distress, communication and specific interventions such as safe storage of medicines. This is one of the most effective ways of helping to reduce the risk of further self-harm or suicide.

The NICE guidelines on self-harm state that initial management should include advising carers of the need to remove all medication or other means of self-harm available to the child or young person who has self-harmed (NICE 2004a). Parents may also need to be more vigilant, not necessarily being with the young person 24 hours a day, but checking that they are okay and observing them on a regular basis.

Managing distress

Some young people can tell their parents or carers when they are struggling. This may include statements about feeling unsafe, or verbal expressions about thoughts and feelings. However, parents sometimes need to be supported to recognise that young people are not easily able to verbalise their distress. Here, other communication systems can be developed and agreed.

Some young people like to use creative ideas like traffic light systems – indicating red, amber or green on their bedroom door to represent if things are going well or if parents need to be worried. Sporty young people may like the football analogy of using red and yellow cards, warning parents that they have fouled or are losing control. Different systems work for different young people, and it does not matter what is used as long as the form of communication is understood by all involved.

Overdoses

We have heard that the large majority of young people who have taken an overdose have done so impulsively with little in the way of prior planning or thought. Things have often built up; young people feel overwhelmed and, faced with the availability of tablets, the act has occurred. This is one of several reasons why we discourage use of the term 'deliberate'. Often, young people do not make a considered decision to self-harm and many believe, rightly or wrongly, that the tablets would do them no harm. In such circumstances, lack of easy access to medicines and other means of self-harm can be a preventative measure. As Anne so powerfully puts it:

> If only the tablets hadn't been there, I would still be the same person I was. Instead I am always going to be a person who has taken an overdose. I will have to live with that for the rest of my life.
>
> Anne, 14

Many parents and young people can see that this approach is a matter of common sense and agree to reduce access to medicines as part of the management plan. However, professionals and parents sometimes challenge the logic of this approach, arguing that the young person can go to the shop and buy tablets if they want to. This is indeed true, but it seems that most do not. This may because it is late at night or they don't want to go out, or they don't want to spend their money on tablets. With barriers to access they may choose to do something else instead. They may call a friend, go on the computer or listen to music, and in doing so, the moment may pass.

Some parents argue that the young person has to learn to take responsibility for themselves. Again, this is true, but we should recognise that many young people struggle to do this, which is why they are self-harming in the first place. Such appraisal by parents can reflect how they are feeling about their child's self-harm. For example, they may be angry with the young person and feel they want to punish them. They may be finding it difficult to show them that they care, when this is often exactly what the young person needs during times of distress.

Cutting

Restricting access to sharp items is less straightforward. Young people use a variety of things to cut themselves including razors, scissors, knives, broken glass, pencil sharpener blades and broken shards of plastic. The principle of harm minimisation should be discussed with parents and carers as well as young people themselves. It is unrealistic and inappropriate to remove everything sharp from the house or environment in which a young person is living. However, there may be specific items that the young person uses to self-harm, and having those removed would help them to resist any urges to cut.

Attention should also be paid to where the self-harm usually occurs. For example, if the young person usually cuts themselves in their bedroom, it makes sense not to keep razors in there.

However, we know from some young people who have cut themselves many times and over long periods of time, that having something available, to hand, clean and not used by other people is important. This may be preferable to them finding and using something dirty such as a piece of broken glass and using this in desperation. So, as strange as it may seem to parents and carers and some professionals, removing all sharp items, even if it was possible, may not be the safest thing to do.

Being there

Simply being with a young person is preventative in itself. Ideally, parents should be able to talk with their son or daughter about thoughts and feelings, but this is not always possible. Communication may be poor, and both young people and adults can struggle with their respective roles in a parent–child relationship where emotional support is required.

It is not uncommon for parents not to know how to approach sensitive issues with their children. Many need support from professionals to build strategies and confidence to communicate effectively, and for some the process can be enormously difficult. However, just being with young people doing everyday things can be sufficient and containing in itself. It is often at night when the young person is alone, not with friends, or less distracted that they are more vulnerable to self-harm.

Sometimes, when young people do confide in a parent, the worries and problems they describe may not seem that serious to the parent. For example, their son or daughter may talk about feeling ugly or stupid, or not fitting in with others at school. Just as it is important to reassure them and tell them how special they are, it is also helpful to empathise with how negative the young person is feeling. This is to accept and validate how they feel and to avoid dismissing their feelings.

Support for parents

A recent study has suggested that young people who do not live with both parents seem to be at increased risk of repetition of self-harm (Anderson *et al.* 2009). The reasons for this are not fully understood. Whilst it may be possible that young people feel some sense of loss or rejection, the parent may also be feeling less supported and more stressed in their parenting role.

When their child is suicidal or self-harming, there are several key issues that are important to parents. Not least is trying to understand why they have self-harmed in the first place, and this has been discussed in earlier chapters. Also is the desire to keep them safe. Another theme is the need for support for themselves. Whilst they may have been supported during the assessment and treatment process, having peer group support is often extremely helpful.

Parent support groups

Parenting support is any activity or facility aimed at providing information, advice and support to parents and carers to help them in bringing up their children. Whilst not routinely available, there is a growing awareness of the important role parent support groups can play in supporting young people who are suicidal or self-harming.

Support groups can help parents and carers to feel less isolated and provide an opportunity to express feelings such as guilt, shame, anger and distress. This is in a forum which provides support from other parents who may be in similar circumstances. The availability of parental support groups will vary depending on where people live.

FLASH (Families Learning about Self-Harm) in Berkshire is an example of a specialist parenting group aimed at parents and carers of children over 11 years old. This is a partnership between specialist CAMHS and universal services providing early intervention, parenting support and guidance for families of children who self-harm (Massie 2008).

Written information

Written information can be helpful in engaging and, therefore, involving parents and carers as well as young people themselves. For example, leaflets can be designed to inform parents about the service they and their child can expect to receive. Written information can also set out the choices available to them, including those related to gender of therapist, venue and models of treatment or therapy. Leaflets should be available that explain self-harm. Some national documents are also available including *Truth Hurts* which includes an appendix for parents (Mental Health Foundation and Camelot Foundation 2006).

Verbal and written feedback

We have seen that parents and carers' involvement in care and treatment decisions is often crucial in supporting young people who are suicidal and self-harming. There are different ways of obtaining feedback from parents and carers, and the method used will depend on what has been agreed about information sharing and the stage the young person is at in their support or treatment.

Notwithstanding issues of consent, ongoing verbal feedback during the course of therapy can be helpful in reviewing the balance of parental involvement and potentially the focus of the work. This tends to be specific, perhaps about the frequency of the sessions, content or a wish to involve a different family member, such as an aunt, uncle or grandparent.

When parents or carers have been directly involved in the care and treatment of their son or daughter it is helpful to get some written feedback of their experience of the service. This is so the service can reflect on whether parents and carers feel listened to, that their views are being considered and that they have been appropriately involved.

Written feedback can help to establish themes which can positively influence service development and improvements. For example, parents and carers often highlight the need for written information, such as leaflets about self-harm, information about pharmacological treatments and any parent support groups available to them. Others report their experiences of stigma in using mental health services. They describe how difficult it can be attending appointments, not knowing what to expect, and being worried that their son or daughter would be disadvantaged by accessing mental health services. Written feedback can be useful in helping to identify gaps in service provision and addressing these in collaboration with parents and carers, managers and commissioners.

Other resources for parents

PAPYRUS, a UK charity committed to the prevention of suicide by children, teenagers and young adults, offers a range of resources that are helpful for both parents and professionals. Their publication *Not Just a Cry for Help* offers the following guidance which can be used by parents and carers. They encourage parents to be ALERT as follows:

- Ask young people how they are feeling
- Listen to them
- Empathise with them
- Reassure them
- Try to give support.

They also advise parents and carers not to PANIC:

- Put young people down or do things that might make them feel worse
- Abandon or reject them in any way
- Nag or intrude
- Ignore what has happened
- Criticise their actions.

Another useful resource is *Help is at Hand*, developed by Hawton and Simkin (2008) in collaboration with PAPYRUS, the Samaritans and other key organisations. It aims to help people bereaved by suicide and other sudden traumatic deaths. The book offers both practical and emotional support, and in some areas, groups have been set up using the book as a template for group work.

Virtual support

Like children and young people, parents and carers need to be able to access support in a range of different ways. Some prefer support from family and friends, and others want professional support. Of course, many require both formal and informal support. There is also a growing number of virtual resources for young people who self-harm and their parents or carers.

Parentline Plus is a national charity that works for and with parents. They recognise that family life can be challenging, and help support parents to do their best. They offer email support, an online community message board and small telephone groups, as well as face-to-face group work in some areas of the country. The workers are all parents and many are volunteers. Their strapline is 'we're here because instructions aren't included'.

Parental mental health

As many as one in four adults experience mental health problems, and many are parents. Depending on the severity of their symptoms, their mental health problems may negatively impact on their parenting. It is important that parents with mental health problems receive the appropriate care and support services that they need in order to fulfil their parental role. Some parents self-harm and many have tried to kill themselves. Some misuse drugs and alcohol, which can also have a detrimental impact on parenting.

Specialist CAMHS are sometimes asked to help a child whose parent or carer is self-harming (Wright and Richardson 2003). This requires close collaboration between CAMHS and adult services, and safeguarding children must be at the centre of all interventions. Children in this situation may be inappropriately fulfilling a 'young carer' role, and the welfare of the child should always be paramount. As with young people, it can take parents time to acknowledge that they have mental health problems and agree to access help.

Summary

Parenting is often described as being the most difficult job in the world and is one that comes without any training. In some circumstances, parents may be struggling to meet their own needs and therefore find it more difficult to meet the emotional and psychological needs of their children. When a young person is self-harming the demands may be even greater. Parents of young people who are suicidal or self-harming invariably need support, and if given this they can help improve the long-term outcomes for their child.

As part of helping children and young people who self-harm we should generally encourage the involvement of parents. In most cases this is fairly straightforward, but on some occasions this may not be in the young person's best interests. For example, some parents are not able to put the needs of their child above their own, or have repeatedly broken trust or let them down. In these circumstances we have to be guided by young people. It may be that as the work and therapeutic relationship develops, they may consider minimal parental involvement and that may gradually increase, depending on the circumstances and their experience of their parents during this time.

9 Service provision and care pathways

Key points:

- Professionals who work with children and young people encounter self-harm in a range of residential and community settings. This includes schools, health services, social services placements and prisons. It is important that they are able to recognise self-harm and ensure that young people can access help from the right person or service at the right time.
- Whilst many young people who self-harm should be supported in frontline services, others require assessment or treatment by targeted or specialist services. The skills and competencies required of professionals and other adults in universal or mainstream services are different to those required in specialist self-harm services.
- Care pathways for young people to reach help and support should be clearly defined and agreed by all stakeholders. They should also be easily accessible and readily understood by all professionals and other adults who work with young people who self-harm.
- Tailored interventions for young people who self-harm are provided by specialist CAMHS which provide assessment and treatment for young people with complex, persistent or serious mental health difficulties. In addition, they provide consultation to professionals and workers in primary services who may be working with suicidal young people or those who self-harm.
- It is important that professionals and other adults who work with young people who self-harm feel appropriately trained. Despite guidance, self-harm remains poorly understood by many professionals and other adults who work with children and young people.
- Providing care and treatment for young people who self-harm can be emotionally demanding for adults who work with them. Organisations providing self-harm services should ensure that staff can access ongoing support and supervision.

Introduction

The full range of resources and interventions needed by young people who self-harm spans the responsibilities of many agencies and services. However, care services, including accident and emergency and mental health services, play the greatest role. People who self-harm often come to health services in crisis and may present with a range of emotions including intense worry, unhappiness and anger. Consequently, they often require mental health as well as physical health care services.

However, it is not only health services that support young people who self-harm. Other statutory and third-sector providers also have a key contribution to make. This chapter discusses interventions in primary services and secondary care services for young people who self-harm, and explores the roles and responsibilities of key workers in community and hospital settings. Good practice in referral, admission and discharge procedures are discussed.

The role of accident and emergency departments

Many children and young people who present to health services following self-harm are admitted to A&E departments (Crawford 1998). This is for assessment and treatment and access to medical and surgical beds if they require emergency treatment or recovery facilities. As well as managing the immediate medical or surgical consequences of self-harm, there is also the need to assess risk prior to discharge.

It is estimated that each year about 19,000 children under 16 are admitted to hospital after attempting suicide (Hawton *et al.* 1996). A one-year survey found that more than 60,000 young people aged 12–24 presented to A&E departments following self-harm, and over half were admitted (Hurry and Storey 1998). Concerns have been raised about the quality of self-harm assessments and care by A&E staff (O'Dwyer *et al.* 1991; Pritchard 1995; Clark *et al.* 2000), which partly led to the development of the NICE guidelines on self-harm.

Young people themselves have complained that many A&E and other health staff can be judgemental, unhelpful and unwilling to understand (Social Care Institute for Excellence 2005). The extract on the following page shows how a young person aged 16 experienced A&E.

NICE guidelines

Current NICE guidelines on self-harm focus on the first 48 hours after a child or young person arrives at hospital following self-harm. This is to ensure that high quality physical, psychological and social assessments are carried out. It is essential that there are protocols and guidelines in place between emergency departments and specialist CAMHS. This is so that young people who have self-harmed can have their needs assessed, including an evaluation of future self-harm or suicide risk. However, despite standards set by NICE and professional bodies, the quality of such protocols and the degree of collaboration and joint working between paediatric and mental health services varies considerably in the UK.

My time at A&E

More often than not, self-harm will eventually land you a seat in A&E with all the caring doctors and nurses (apologies to any A&E staff etc, this is based on my own experiences and I appreciate, somewhat like self-harmers, that you're not all to be tarred with the same brush).

Medically trained and compassionate, you'd expect some warmth and understanding at least from here. You'd expect the same level of care as anyone else who passed through the red doors and through the cramped waiting room. All injuries that need treatment should be given the same quality of care, regardless of how the injury was sustained. Yet you believe that because we were the cause we should either 'deal with it' ourselves or be subjected to sub-standard care and punishment resembling treatment.

Would an obese, sedentary male suffering from a heart attack be turned away because they 'did it themselves'?

I've heard stories of wounds being stitched minus the apparently 'optional' anaesthetic because you think we 'don't feel pain'. When I attempted suicide earlier in the year by overdose, my blood pressure was checked on arrival and I was shut in a room until the psychiatrist and my parents came to get me. The only contact I got was when my bed was pulled from the wall when I began to bang my head against it. This resulted in concussion, a rather hefty lump, which again wasn't monitored, and the threat of security and police when I escaped into the outside road and was carried kicking and screaming back into my room.

Appreciated is the fact that A&E staff are overworked, and accepted is the fact that in the agitated depressive state I was in, further exacerbated by the tablets, I was perhaps deemed as a nuisance, but I was out of control.

I was distressed and they shut me in a room for two hours. My experience definitely wasn't an isolated incident, but neither was the genuinely compassionate and caring treatment I'd received at other times in other A&E departments.

My GP, for example, has always closed and cleaned wounds when I haven't been able to make it to A&E. He's talked to me. He's never judged me, and while I do moan about some of the stuff he says, he's been there throughout this whole sorry mess and has given up his own time to help me.

Positive engagement

Attendance at A&E is often the first port of call for a young person who has self-harmed. Treating the physical injuries caused by self-harm in a sensitive, non-stigmatising and non-judgemental manner is an important first step in encouraging them to engage with support services (NSPCC 2009). Children and young people who have attended emergency departments following self-harm should be treated with the same care, respect and privacy as any other patient. This is regardless of the apparent purpose of the self-harm, and health care professionals should take full account of the likely associated distress experienced by young people (NICE 2004a).

Triage

In order to ensure that young people receive an assessment of their self-harm and are able to access appropriate treatment, NICE recommends that a process of triage should be used. Various models of triage exist, including the Australian Triage Scale (ATS) which can be used to assess clinical risk and urgency for treatment. Children and young people's triage doctors and nurses should be trained in the assessment and early management of mental health problems and, in particular, in the assessment and early management of children and young people who have self-harmed. Young people should also be assessed and treated in a separate children's area of the emergency department (NICE 2004a). This is in order to help ensure that care and treatment is developmentally appropriate, and that young people feel welcome.

The Royal College of Psychiatrists (RCP) has produced council reports related to managing self-harm in young people (RCP 1998). Among other things, RCP recommends that young people who self-harm should be admitted to general hospital, since the annual rate of repetition is higher for adolescents who are not admitted (Hawton and Fagg 1992). Discharge from hospital and referral to specialist services should be based on an overall assessment of psychosocial needs and risk.

How do children get referred to specialist services?

We have heard that most young people who self-harm do not come to the attention of professional services and only a minority are assessed by self-harm specialists. However, it is important to point out that not all young people who access specialist services find them acceptable or helpful (Young *et al.* 2007).

Specialist interventions for young people who self-harm are provided by professionals in Tier 2, 3 or 4 CAMHS. Specialist CAMHS provide assessment and treatment services for young people with complex, persistent or serious self-harm. In addition, they also provide consultation to professionals and workers in primary services who may be working with suicidal young people or those who self-harm (Wright and Richardson 2003).

The tiered model of service delivery

The Health Advisory Service (1995) review report, *Together We Stand*, gave a detailed account of the characteristics of nationwide CAMHS, with sections on epidemiology, needs assessment, service principles, and service commissioning and provision. The report promoted the national adaptation of the acronym CAMHS and with its framework of four tiers, helped promote the important message that child and adolescent mental health is everyone's business.

The CAMHS tiered model of service delivery is a framework to organise the commissioning, management and delivery of mental health services for children and young people with mental health problems and disorders (Health Advisory Service 1995). This framework is currently the preferred model for planning and delivering child mental health services which often includes self-harm services. Although the framework has been in place for nearly 15 years, it is, however, sometimes misunderstood by service users, commissioners and providers (see Figure 9.1).

Tier 1

Parents and frontline professionals in primary services are usually the first to recognise self-harm. These include GPs, teachers, health visitors and school nurses. Sometimes referred to as universal, frontline or primary services, Tier 1 services are those in which children receive day-to-day care, education or health care interventions. Such services include those provided in schools, GP practices and children's homes, and professionals in these settings should have a basic understanding about self-harm, and know how to refer a child for primary care or more specialist assessments.

Professionals in Tier 1 services are most likely to encounter young people who self-harm in the context of interpersonal difficulties, such as those arising from bullying or problems within the family. An awareness of self-harm may enable Tier 1 professionals to contextualise a young person's behaviour and help them continue to provide frontline services for this vulnerable group. In order for Tier 1 professionals to most effectively meet the needs of young people who self-harm, they require training and support. This training may be most effectively targeted at services which have children and young people with higher rates of self-harm. As we saw earlier, this includes looked after children, children who have been abused and young people in secure settings.

The NICE guidelines on self-harm recommend that primary care workers should assess the urgent physical and mental health needs of young people who have self-harmed during the previous 48-hour period (NICE 2004a). In the case of self-poisoning, primary care workers should refer the young person to A&E and also consider referral for other forms of self-harm, such as cutting. Referral of a young person to A&E will depend on the severity, intention, and frequency of the self-harm.

| **Tier 1** |
| Services at primary level by professionals providing non-specialist CAMHS in health, education, social services and youth justice settings. This involves mental health promotion, early identification of mental health problems and, in some cases, treatment for less severe mental health problems, e.g. sleep, temper tantrums, behaviour problems at home/school and bereavement |
| **Professionals** |
| Health visitors, practice nurses, school nurses, SureStart worker, GPs, voluntary sector workers, youth workers, teachers, Healthy Schools Project workers, social workers, family support workers |

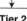

| **Tier 2** |
| Individual professionals who work relatively independently from other services, but relate to each other through a network. They provide training and consultation to Tier 1 workers, outreach to identify complex, severe or persistent mental disorders and signpost children and young people to specialist CAMHS at Tiers 2 or 3 |
| **Professionals** |
| Clinical psychologist, educational psychologist, child and adolescent psychiatrist, YOT, health nurse specialist, primary mental health worker, community paediatrician, hospital paediatrician |

Most children with mental health problems will be seen at Tiers 1 and 2

| **Tier 3** |
| Specialist multidisciplinary child and adolescent teams |
| **Professionals** |
| Psychiatrists, mental health nurses, psychologists, social workers, family therapists and others providing assessment and treatment for children and young people with complex, persistent or severe mental disorders. Assessment for referrals to Tier 4. Provision of support and training for Tier 2 and offer consultation to Tier 1 professionals. |

| **Tier 4** |
| Specialist multidisciplinary child and adolescent teams. Inpatient child and adolescent units may also have support from occupational therapists, speech and language therapists and creative therapists who specialise in art, music, drama or play therapy. |

| Inpatient child and adolescent units, day services | Intensive home based treatment teams/crisis outreach services | Outpatient services for eating disorders, neuropsychiatric problems, sexual abuse, OCD, etc. |

Figure 9.1 NHS Health Advisory tiered model of CAMHS service delivery (1995) (from McDougall (2006)

Sometimes, referral to A&E is not made as the assessment of risk by the primary worker is low, and their needs can be met more appropriately elsewhere. Where primary workers suspect that a young person is harming themselves, they should consider discussing this with a colleague in a specialist CAMHS team. This may result in a formal consultation and the referral of the young person for a specialist CAMHS assessment (Armstrong 2006).

Tier 2

Tier 2 services are provided by professionals with additional training or expertise in child and adolescent mental health. The role of a Tier 2 professional is to provide direct assessment or treatment interventions for individual children and young people with less complex problems than those requiring Tier 3 or 4 services, and to offer support, guidance and training for Tier 1 professionals providing frontline services. Tier 2 professionals sometimes support young people who are self-harming to develop low intensity skills interventions, often focusing on emotional regulation and the development of alternatives to self-harm as coping strategies.

Professionals working in services at Tiers 1 and 2 must be able to access specialist CAMHS. This is where they have concerns that a child or young person they are working with may require a full multidisciplinary assessment or specialist treatment for their self-harming or suicidal behaviour. Young people presenting with repeated self-harm should always be referred to Tier 3 CAMHS for assessment. Referral to social services either using section 47 (Child Protection) or section 17 (Child in Need) of the Children Act 1989 may also be required if there are significant concerns about family functioning and the welfare of the child or young person.

Tier 3

Tier 3 services are dedicated multidisciplinary specialist teams providing comprehensive assessment, treatment and consultation services for children and young people with complex, persistent or severe mental health needs and disorders. Many referrals to Tier 3 CAMHS are of suicidal children and young people and those who self-harm (McDougall and Crocker 2001). Tier 3 teams usually comprise nurses, psychiatrists, psychologists, family therapists, social workers and therapists. They offer a range of treatments for suicidal or self-harming young people, including individual and group therapy.

Tier 3 CAMHS usually provide specialist assessments of self-harm and suicidal behaviour by using a rota. This means that clinicians can assess a young person in crisis and waiting times are reduced.

Tier 4

Sometimes young people have very complex, severe or debilitating mental disorders and they cannot be safely or effectively managed by Tier 3 CAMHS. Tier 4 services are highly specialised tertiary CAMHS and include inpatient child and adolescent units, specialised eating disorder services and forensic CAMHS, as well as multi-agency services, such as home treatment services, community support teams and crisis teams. The evidence base for Tier 4 services is in its infancy (McDougall *et al.* 2007).

Inpatient mental health admission

The large majority of young people who self-harm are not treated in hospital. Factors warranting consideration for admission include acute suicidality associated with mental disorder, and high risk behaviour which cannot safely be managed by the family or community based services.

Most admissions to Tier 4 inpatient settings happen 'informally'. This means either that the child or young person has agreed to come into hospital and accept help with their mental health problems, or their parent has consented. This is important since commitment to receiving help is linked to better outcomes for this group. On other occasions, where the young person does not recognise or agree that they require hospital admission, and the risks are such they can not remain at home, the Mental Health Act 1983 may be used to provide compulsion and admit young people to hospital against their wishes. This is discussed further in Chapter 11.

Inpatient units providing assessment and treatment for self-harming or suicidal young people should have a clearly defined and structured treatment programme and a team with the ability to tolerate and take therapeutic risks. This includes the capacity to discharge young people who remain at risk of self-harm or suicide if admission is ineffective or makes a young person's self-harming worse.

What are the risks of hospital admission?

Admission to a child or adolescent mental health inpatient setting would not usually be to manage self-harm per se, but would be to contain associated risks or address additional mental health co-morbidity, such as psychosis or depression. Indeed, some argue that admitting self-harming young people to hospital may often be ineffective or even make their self-harm worse. Health professionals sometimes try and stop young people self-harming. This removes power and control and may create the very circumstances that led to the self-harm in the first place.

In addition, the social contagion theory described earlier in the book suggests that some young people may learn self-harming behaviour from others. The NICE guidelines on depression in children and young people warn that an impressionable child or young person with high levels of self-harming behaviour is at risk of acquiring additional dysfunctional behaviours or coping strategies, even where a skilled and experienced staff team openly address such potential difficulties (National Collaborating Centre for Mental Health 2005).

It is therefore important to pay close attention to the mix of young people on the child or adolescent inpatient unit at any one time. Caring for and treating young people who self-harm along with young people who may be acutely psychotic could be counterproductive. This is because both groups of young people require different treatment programmes and benefit from different therapeutic milieus. Young people who self-harm often require a busy arousing programme of activity and frequently engage in group activities. By contrast, those who are psychotic often require a low stimulus environment and individual treatments (Cotgrove *et al.* 2007).

Managing transitions

Many young people who harm themselves stop doing so without professional intervention. Others recover with support from adults who understand and can help. Some, however, continue to require ongoing support with their self-harm as they leave adolescence and enter adulthood. Whilst some young people experience a smooth transition from adolescent to adult services, others find the process anxiety-provoking and stressful. Their self-harm may increase as a result.

It is of concern that various reports have confirmed that transitional arrangements for young people who self-harm are often poorly defined, crisis led and frequently managed on a case-to-case basis (Singh 2009). These have included *Turned Upside Down*, a three-year study by the Mental Health Foundation which focused on the views of 45 young people aged between 16 and 25. The report showed that young people found neither children's nor adult's services adequate in terms of supporting them during transition (Smith and Leon 2001).

Research shows that many young people 'fall through the net' due to inadequate and fragmented mental health services, and poorly developed care pathways and transitions between CAMHS and adult mental health services (Pugh *et al.* 2006). Dedicated 16–19 services are not available in all areas of the country, and this leaves gaps in access for many young people (McDougall *et al.* 2009).

It is not only transitions from children's to adult's services that young people who self-harm require support with. There is well documented evidence that the transition from junior school to secondary school; or the process of leaving college to start employment can be stressful events for many children and young people. During this transition, one-to-one teacher support decreases and the demands placed by a bigger peer group increases. Self-harm can often be a manifestation of the difficulties children and young people are facing and struggling with.

Innovative services

Although there is no compelling evidence that specialist self-harm services reduce repetition rates, they have been found to reduce the need for hospital admission (Kapur *et al.* 2002; Taylor *et al.* 2006). One example of a specialist service for young people who self-harm is the Adolescent Self-Harm service in Glasgow. This is a rapid intervention, home based service based on CBT.

Another example of a specialist service is the Oxford Looked After Children Dialectical Behaviour Therapy team. This is also an NSF Development initiative aimed at children with complex needs, including self-harm or suicidal behaviour, and who are difficult to engage. The project aims to help young people who self-harm change their lifestyles and avoid hospital admission (Massie 2008).

The Nottingham Self-Harm team is another example of an innovative service, led by a nurse consultant to provide hospital assessments and follow-up for young people who self-harm.

Hartlepool Self-Harm Service

A further innovative development is the Hartlepool Self-Harm Service. Funded by the Children's National Service Framework development initiatives for psychological well-being and mental health, this is a partnership between specialist CAMHS and children's services, providing an early intervention service for school-age children and young people who self-harm. The initiative builds on capacity in schools to assist in recognition, response and management of self-harm. It also aims to improve access to services before the young person reaches crisis, reducing the number of young people presenting at accident and emergency departments.

Protocols have been agreed between the team and local hospital. If a young person presents at A&E with self-harm they will be admitted to the paediatric ward if they are under 16. If they are over 16, overnight admission for medical and mental health assessment is encouraged, but some young people refuse and decide to go home. In this situation, the CAMHS team will follow them up the next day.

The Hartlepool project has also developed the Vulnerability Assessment Screening Tool (VAST), which is used by school teachers to recognise and address behaviours which are of concern, including cutting. The project has not yet evaluated service user data, but, interestingly, its needs analysis did not show a wide variation between the self-harming behaviour of girls and boys (Massie 2008).

Self-harm protocols

The aim of a protocol is to improve the quality of support, guidance and advice provided by staff who are working with young people who self-harm.

Protocols for self-harm focus on clinical interventions and care pathways, and set standards for assessment, care and treatment (NICE 2004a).

The majority of self-harm protocols summarise care pathways, define referral criteria, and set out roles and responsibilities of professionals in contact with young people who self-harm. Most protocols for self-harm are multi-agency agreements. They often identify a single point of referral or entry to a service, set thresholds for accessing treatment interventions and include 'signposts' where referral to another agency may be required, for example, due to the severity or risks associated with a young person's self-harm. Figures 9.2 and 9.3 are two examples of self-harm protocols. It is important that pathways to services for young people are clear and developed as part of multi-agency agreements and children's services plans.

Quality standards

The Royal College of Psychiatrists has published quality standards for health care professionals focused on improving services for people who self-harm (Royal College of Psychiatrists 2006). Funded by the Health Foundation, these have been developed in conjunction with a range of professional bodies and organisations including the British Association for Emergency Medicine and the College of Emergency Medicine; the Royal College of Nursing and the National Collaborating Centre for Mental Health. Service user experts were also consulted. The standards are intended to support emergency department staff, ambulance service, mental health teams and primary care practitioners. The quality standards for self-harm are mapped against the Department of Health (2006), with clear references to the Commission's core standards focusing on standards of services that all patients should be able to expect

The standards apply to people of all ages, but include specific criteria on children and young people aged under 16 (see Table 9.1).

Telephone support lines

In 2007, ChildLine received over half a million calls and over 175,000 children were counselled. Over 6,000 of the callers talked about self-harm, many of whom were already engaged with public services but whose needs were not being fully met (NSPCC 2009). This illustrates the demand for telephone helplines for children and young people in crisis. The National Inquiry report into self-harm by young people suggested that telephone lines may be a common source of help because they offer consistent, non-judgemental advice, and that some control can be maintained by the caller (Mental Health Foundation and Camelot Foundation 2006). However, there have also been critics of telephone support lines, claiming that they are a poor substitute for face-to-face help.

Derby multi-agency self-harm pathway

A child/young person tells you that they have self-harmed or expressed suicidal thoughts	A child/young person tells you that they have self-harmed or expressed suicidal thoughts

If self-harm took place **within the last 48 hours** and involves ingestion, serious lacerations or excessive dose/omission of prescribed medication	If self-harm took place **longer than 48 hours ago** and involves ingestion, serious lacerations or excessive dose/omission of prescribed medication

• Child/young person should be taken to hospital emergency department • Discuss with your manager/safeguarding colleague • Ensure own support • Consider contacting parent/carer • Document in keeping with agency procedure	Contact any of the following: • GP • NHS Direct • A&E • Children's A&E

• Clarify who is best placed to talk with the child/young person. If this is a re-occurring situation, ensure a consistent person/s deals with incident
• Indicate willingness to talk to child or young person about self harm
• Try to be non-judgemental
• Validate their feelings
• Go at child's pace
• Confidentiality: tell them who you will pass information to and how
• Assess situation re safety, mental health, context, risk and resilience factors in relation to Common Assessment Framework
• Is there an immediate risk management issue? If so, speak with your manager and consider seeking consultation from safeguarding colleague/CAMHS or social care.
• Do you feel the self-harm arises from the child's life context? If so, discuss with safeguarding colleague and refer to social care
• Do you feel the young person may be mentally unwell? If so, consider urgent referral to Specialist CAMHS
• Discuss with manager/safeguarding colleague/ school community nurse as appropriate
• Consider parent/carer contact
• Document in keeping with agency procedure

Figure 9.2 Derby multi-agency self-harm pathway

Source: Derby City Partnership multi-agency self-harm protocol

Figure 9.3 Nottinghamshire and Nottingham city self-harm care pathway

NOTTINGHAMSHIRE & NOTTINGHAM CITY SELF-HARM CARE PATHWAY
What to do if you are concerned about a young person self-harming

Tier 1 Universal Services	Tier 2 Targeted Services	Tier 3 Specialist Services	Tier 4 Highly Specialist Services
Low level risk self-harm Superficial, minor self-harm in stable social context. Some indicators of good emotional health, functioning well. No evidence of suicidal intent. Good support networks.	**Repeated and more worrying self-harm behaviour** More frequent or severe self-harm. More pervasive stressors, poorer coping strategies and fluctuating mental health. SH that presents alongside mild–moderate MH problems e.g. depression and trauma.	**Persistent and severe self-harm** More complex, frequent, high risk behaviours – concerns re isolation, substance misuse, suicidal intent. SH that presents alongside moderate–severe MH problems e.g. depression and trauma. Poor support / protective factors.	**High risk suicidal behaviour** Concerns about severe mental health disorder, where risk can not be managed in community.

What action should you take?

Promotion of healthy ways of expressing emotions. Talk to YP, ideally encourage parental involvement. Self-help information, coping strategies. If situation deteriorates seek consultation and support from Tier 2 and possible referral, via CAF.	Continue working with YP, gather info, involve network around the YP. Assess and monitor risk. If situation deteriorates inform YP worried – may need additional support, consultation, joint working or referral to Tier 3 via single point of access. Access consultation via Self-Harm Team or Tier 3 EDT (Emotional Disorders Team).	Work with YP on agreed plan, access clinical supervision and MDT support. Monitor risk and review progress. If situation deteriorates consider Tier 4 assessment.	Assess and develop management plan for mental health and suicidal behaviour. Involve and transfer to Tier 3 when risk reduced assessment / treatment complete.

Services and help available....

UNIVERSAL School nurse, youth workers, GP, schools, Connexions PA Base 51 – Counselling Speak Easy	**TARGETED** MALTS, DEHWT Compass LD / CAMHS Early Intervention Service Community Paediatricians YOTs	**SPECIALIST** Self-Harm Team EDT (Emotional Disorders Team) H2H (Head 2 Head) CLA (Children Looked After)	**HIGHLY SPECIALIST** Adolescent Unit

Monitor and document concerns, seek appropriate supervision and involvement of line manager.
IN THE CASE OF AN EMERGENCY REFER YOUNG PERSON TO THEIR GP OR HOSPITAL EMERGENCY DEPARTMENT IMMEDIATELY
YP under 16 who attend emergency department for self-harm will be admitted and assessed by Tier 3 CAMHS. 16- and 17-year-olds will be assessed by Adult Mental Health Services and referred to CAMHS (EDT) for follow-up.

Table 9.1 Adapted from Royal College of Psychiatrists *Quality Standards for Healthcare Professionals*

Standard	Criterion
Appropriately trained children's nurses or doctors should be available to ensure that young people who have self-harmed are:	• Triaged by appropriately trained children's nurses • Assessed by appropriately trained children's doctors or nurses • Treated by appropriately trained doctors or nurses
Young people should be provided with facilities and information which is child friendly:	• Young people should be triaged, assessed and treated in a separate children's area of the emergency department • Written information provided to young people should be written in child-friendly language
Young people who have self-harmed should be admitted to an age-appropriate environment:	• Children and young people who have self-harmed should normally be admitted overnight to a paediatric ward • Children and young people should be assessed fully the following day, before discharge or further treatment is initiated • Alternative placements should be available depending on the age of the child, family circumstances, the time of presentation to services, safeguarding issues, and the physical and mental health of the child. This might include admission to a child or adolescent psychiatric inpatient unit where necessary • For young people aged over 14 admission to a ward for adolescents may be considered if this is available and preferred by the young person • A paediatrician should normally have overall responsibility for the treatment and care of children and young people who have been admitted to a paediatric ward following self-harm
All assessment and treatment of young people should be conducted with the appropriate consent:	• Following admission of a child or young person who has self-harmed, the admitting team should obtain parental (or other legally responsible adult) consent for the mental health assessment of the child or young person
Staff who have emergency contact with young people who have self-harmed should have received training in:	• Assessing mental capacity and consent • The concept of Gillick competence • Safeguarding vulnerable children • Recognition of abuse • Confidentiality issues related to children and young people • Use of the Mental Health Act, Mental Capacity Act and the Children Act • Assessing risk in young people
CAMHS professionals who are involved in the assessment and treatment of children and young people who have self-harmed should:	• Work specifically with children and young people and their families or carers after self-harm • Have regular supervision • Have access to consultation with senior colleagues

continued

Table 9.1 Adapted from Royal College of Psychiatrists Quality Standards for Healthcare
Professionals, *continued*

Standard	Criterion
Children and young people admitted to a paediatric ward following self-harm should be assessed appropriately:	• All children and young people who have self-harmed should be assessed by health care professionals experienced in the assessment of children and adolescents • Assessment should include a full assessment of the family, their social situation and any child protection issues
Young people who have self-harmed (and their carers) should be offered appropriate advice and treatment:	• Initial management should include advising parents or carers of the need to remove all medications or other means of self-harm available • For young people who have self-harmed several times, consideration may be given to offering developmental group psychotherapy with other young people who have repeatedly self-harmed. This should include at least six sessions. Extension of the group therapy may also be offered. The precise length of this should be decided jointly by the service user and clinician

PAPYRUS is a voluntary UK organisation committed to the prevention of
suicide and the promotion of mental health and emotional well-being. It
offers support for those dealing with suicide, depression or emotional distress
– particularly teenagers and young adults. They operate a confidential telephone helpline offering support, practical advice and information to young
people as well as their family, friends and professionals.

Is self-harm guidance effective?

It is important to remember that guidelines are not a substitute for professional knowledge, experience or expertise. Rather, they complement good
practice and, like all guidelines, have their limitations. There seems to be little doubt that clinical guidelines, parameters and protocols generally improve
clinical practice (Hill and Taylor 2001). Guidance such as that published by
the National Collaborating Centre on behalf of NICE has been developed
from empirical evidence, the clinical consensus of experts and the voice of
service users. They set standards or principles in relation to good practice
based on the best available evidence.

A review of protocols for the management of self-harm by young people
revealed that many services fail to implement good practice recommendations
(Dorer 1998). These findings are consistent with the research of Armstrong
(1995) who explored the management of young people who self-harm. In this
study, nine hospital departments and six GP practices were asked about their
referral and treatment guidelines. The study found that only four services had
formal guidelines.

Although National guidelines were published at the time, it is important
to note that both studies described above were conducted over ten years ago.

In the last decade, substantial guidance has been issued and quality standards are now available. Therefore, it is hoped that practice is improving and young people are receiving better services from health care professionals. However, the messages from young people throughout this book suggest that there is still a way to go.

Training

Everyone shares a responsibility to promote positive mental health and well-being within their role. It is important that professionals and other adults who work with young people who self-harm feel appropriately trained. Despite guidance, self-harm is poorly understood by many professionals and other adults who work with children and young people.

The NICE guidelines on self-harm highlight the need for training across the workforce and make several recommendations and good practice points (NICE 2004a). Improving staff knowledge and attitudes is the key to better services and reduction in the substantial morbidity and mortality associated with self-harm. The guidelines state that clinical and non-clinical staff who have contact with people in any setting should be provided with appropriate training to equip them to understand and care for people who have self-harmed (NICE 2004a).

In particular, emergency departments should make training available in the assessment of mental health needs and the preliminary management of mental health problems, for all staff working in that environment. In addition, mental health services and emergency department services should jointly develop regular training programmes in the psychosocial assessment and early management of self-harm, to be undertaken by all health care professionals who may assess or treat people who have self-harmed.

The National Inquiry into self-harm by young people found that health, education and social care professionals were not receiving the training or guidance they needed to support young people who self-harm (Mental Health Foundation and Camelot Foundation 2006). The report of the Inquiry recommended that a comprehensive self-harm strategy requires both a broad, generic focus on promoting positive well being, and behaviour-specific information, training and intervention.

As well as formal training in the assessment and management of self-harm and suicidal behaviour, there is much to be learnt from taking the opportunity to work alongside and 'shadow' experienced colleagues, and to develop skills through supervised experience.

Supervision

Working with young people who are suicidal or self-harming is an emotive and challenging area of work. It is crucial that all professionals and other adults have access to support and supervision (Best 2005). When assessing and working with young people who self-harm, discussion of one's concerns with colleagues is an essential part of good practice. There needs to be both formal and informal support structures in place and access to regular clinical supervision. This enables space for the reflection of the work on one's own feelings but also aids the development of high quality clinical assessments and practice. A good rule of thumb is that when a young person cannot manage their own feelings, it is very important that their carers are equipped to manage their own.

Lyon (1997) suggests that three risks face professionals who are caring for suicidal or self-harming young people (see Table 9.2).

It is therefore important that the risks to professionals when working with young people who are suicidal or self-harming are recognised, managed and addressed. It is vital that professional boundaries are defined and maintained, that the professional is aware of their own responses to a young person in distress, and that organisations have systems in place to provide supervision, support and training.

Advocacy

Sometimes young people who are suicidal or self-harming do not want their parents involved or do not find their involvement helpful. Other times parents do not involve themselves or feel out of their depth. Either way, young people can be left feeling alone and advocacy can be very helpful. This is not to say that advocacy is an alternative to parental involvement. Although there are different types of advocates, in general they work as volunteers or paid

Table 9.2 Risks facing professionals (adapted from Lyon 1997)

Risk	Reason
Staff may be challenged	Young people often challenge adults as part of establishing their own identities. At a time of experiencing rapid change and confusion themselves, young people may sometimes enter into confrontations and conflict with professionals.
Staff may be rejected	Young people who are distressed may feel compelled to repeat past experiences. If they have previously been abused or rejected, they may reject first. Sometimes, the closer they get to an adult the more worrying this feels. In this situation, the professional should be consistent and steady, but not intrusive.
Staff may get over involved	Vulnerable young people may be suspicious and wary of forming relationships with professionals. They may be seeking trust, understanding and warmth. It can be difficult to maintain boundaries with young people who are self-harming or suicidal. Within a confiding and close relationship it is easy for the professional to feel that they are the only one able to deal with the young person's problems. This is a common, seductive and sometimes frightening experience for professionals.

workers who have been trained in listening and negotiating skills. Their role is to respect the views and wishes of the person they advocate for, promoting their rights to access information, services and opportunities (MIND 2009). Jo is an advocate who works with young people in hospital (see extract below).

My role as an advocate – Jo

My son was 15 years old when he was admitted to a mental health unit and our lives as a family changed dramatically over a short space of time. My days consisted of visiting my son, attending meetings about his future care and spending hours researching, trying to increase my knowledge and understanding of mental health problems, whilst also trying to maintain normality for my daughter who was only one year old at the time.

Ultimately, I lost my job, my partner left and I had to sell our home. I didn't know who to turn to, friends and family didn't seem to know what to say and at that time I didn't know anyone else who was going through similar circumstances. I had never felt so alone in my life. My son at this time had all but given up and I worried about how we would get through this as a family. We were allocated a family therapist from the adolescent unit, she listened and gave us an opportunity to offload all our fears and frustrations, and she gave us greater understanding of the services available which enabled me to access support that met my son's needs. In short, she gave us hope.

My son eventually came home. The relief was enormous but because he had been in hospital for so long we had to go right back to basics. We had fantastic support from CAMHS and I am delighted to say he is doing really well.

Although it was a truly traumatic experience for my family, it was also an important learning curve for us. Over the last four years I have attained a good knowledge of the services that are available, and have become aware of the difficulties young people have in accessing them. I have never forgotten the difference it made to us when somebody listened and what we were able to achieve because of it. I knew I wanted to give something back and felt very passionately about becoming involved in some way. I therefore decided to start up and provide an advocacy service for young people with mental health problems.

I now meet with young people on a regular basis, slowly building trusting relationships and trying to address any issues they may have. I soon realised that self-harm was a reoccurring issue. The young people I support explain that self-harm is a way of releasing tension and pain when they feel there is nobody to listen or understand how they were feeling. I believe that by listening, providing support and information and encouraging young people to speak up, they are empowered to obtain the individual care and services they need. Advocacy helps young people address their own issues and enables personal growth and recovery.

The feedback I have received for the advocacy service has been very positive. The following quotes have been provided by parents and young people who have used the service.

'I found the advocacy service very supportive to myself and my daughter. It was reassuring to know that a person independent of the staff had a professional overview of what was happening.'

'An invaluable service, it is great being able to speak to someone who has been through similar circumstances, feeling there is hope even when you feel low.'

'It was great to have a listening ear, it relieved pressure, allowing me to deal with issues in a different way rather than hurting myself.'

'It is so easy to talk to Jo, which is good as you feel comfortable and confident speaking about your issues.'

'Jo takes the time to listen, she understands and helps me a lot. She helps me talk to other staff and to get what I want and deserve.'

'My advocate helped me apply for benefits I didn't know I was entitled to, which will help me get out and about a bit more when I get home.'

Summary

Wherever possible, models for care, treatment and service delivery should be based on evidence and established best practice guidelines. Various guidelines exist to assist clinicians, commissioners and managers in planning, delivering and evaluating self-harm services. Yet all too often, the services that children and families receive do not reflect best practice.

In the UK, guidelines published by the National Institute for Clinical Excellence describe evidence-based interventions and models of service provision which are known to produce positive outcomes. Health professionals and others should consult these best practice guidelines at every stage of the assessment and treatment process.

10 Preventing suicide and self-harm

A public health priority

Key points:

- Self-harm by young people places economic demands on health and social care services. Public health strategies that focus on universal interventions to prevent and reduce self-harm by children and young people may offset the future burden on paediatric, mental health and social services.
- Preventing self-harm and suicide requires a comprehensive, integrated effort involving children and young people, families and communities, schools and the media. No single approach is likely to be effective in addressing what is a large-scale universal problem.
- School-based interventions offer the potential to improve outcomes for children and young people who self-harm by promoting emotional health and well-being and intervening early. School-based professionals are in key positions to support young people who self-harm or feel suicidal, and refer those who may require specialist assessment or treatment to specialist services.
- Young people who self-harm, as well as their parents and carers, siblings and friends, are affected by stigma. Just as stress can build up in a young person who has no appropriate source of support, so too can it negatively impact on their social networks. Reducing the stigma associated with self-harm should be a key part of all that we do as health professionals.
- Campaigns to promote awareness, recognition and understanding about self-harm are crucial if the helping and caring professions and wider public are to improve outcomes for young people who self-harm.
- Several training packages are available to help health professionals become more knowledgeable and skilled in assessing and working with young people who self-harm.
- There are a growing number of online resources for children and young people who self-harm. Whilst many focus on recovery, advice and support and offer the potential to highlight positive messages about self-harm, others reinforce negative messages and promote self-harm in an unhelpful way.

Background

Self-harm and attempted suicide have been steadily increasing since the 1960s and are presently a serious public health concern (Centers for Disease Control 1992; Schmidtke *et al.* 1996; Hawton *et al.* 1996; Kerfoot 2000; Fox and Hawton 2004). This is not only in Western societies; research in developing countries has also shown that self-harm is reaching epidemic proportions and is a public health priority across the globe (Eddleston *et al.* 1998).

Suicide is a leading cause of death among young people (Windfhur 2008), and we have previously seen that young people who self-harm represent the highest risk group for subsequent suicide (Hawton 1992). High rates of self-harm and suicidal behaviour are often a result of war, poverty, poor human rights, social deprivation and lack of opportunities for young people.

Whilst some countries have implemented national suicide prevention strategies based on guidance from the UN and WHO, many have not and suicide prevention is not defined as an explicit health priority (Windfhur 2009).

The emotional health and well-being of British children and young people

Mental health promotion strategies aim to encourage a positive view of mental health rather than highlighting disorders, illnesses or deficits. This is with the purpose of developing the building blocks to emotional health and well-being, such as self-esteem, conflict resolution skills and the ability to face and manage the challenges of growing up. However, whilst holistic, multi-dimensional self-esteem based programmes have been found to have positive impacts on young people's emotional health and well-being, their impact on reducing self-harm and suicide is yet to be demonstrated (NHS Health Development Agency 2004).

Despite good evidence, the focus on mental health promotion and early intervention should be stronger and better specified in UK policy. When we consider self-harm, support and treatment at an earlier stage is likely to be more effective and less costly than that which will be needed over a lifetime if the opportunity for prevention and early intervention is missed.

We have heard that adolescence is often a difficult period to navigate, even in the most favourable of circumstances. However, recent research claims that British teenagers are among the unhappiest in the world (UNICEF 2007). The report shows that Britain is in the bottom third in five of the six categories, making Britain's children unhappier and feeling less loved than those in almost any of the world's wealthiest nations.

Investing to save

The emotional health and well-being of children and young people should be of major concern to world leaders. The future prosperity of our planet and its inhabitants depends crucially on the future welfare of our children. Recent national children's policy and research reports highlight the need for early intervention to prevent problems during childhood (Department of Health 2004; Action for Children and New Economics Foundation 2009; Gunnell *et al.* 2009).

Failure to interrupt the negative developmental trajectories of children places a future burden on the economy through long-term demands on adult mental health services, social services, general health services and the criminal justice system. In the current financial climate, it is more important than ever for services to get it right first time for children and young people. The King's Fund has projected that the cost of mental health services will increase from £22.5 billion in 2007 to at least £32.6 billion by 2026. If we add loss of earnings and the costs that fall to other agencies, this figure will be even higher.

The *Backing the Future* report by Action for Children and the New Economics Foundation suggests that the costs to the UK economy of failing to tackle family breakdown, substance misuse and mental disorder may cost as much as £4 trillion over two decades (Action for Children and New Economics Foundation 2009). We know that these are all potent risk factors for self-harm and suicide. The report goes on to say that providing early interventions to prevent psychosocial problems could save the UK economy £486 billion over 20 years. They recommend moving to a social return on investment, which helps services understand and manage the social and economic value they are creating (Action for Children and New Economics Foundation 2009).

How can the problem be addressed?

It is notoriously difficult to accurately predict those young people who self-harm who later go on to kill themselves (Kapur *et al.* 2004b). Follow-up studies in the past few decades have usually been between five and ten years post intervention. Earlier studies have had a much longer duration but may not reflect the major changes in epidemiological factors in self-harm and completed suicide rates (Hawton and Catalan 1987).

The socio-economic factors that combine to produce self-harm, such as poverty and educational disadvantage, and the problems which are associated with these, such as alcohol and substance misuse, domestic violence and mental illness, are each universal prevention priorities. Preventing this negative sequelae and intervening early in childhood may reduce rates of self-harm in adulthood.

Evidence from WHO shows that factors preventing young people from self-harm and suicide include effective coping skills, positive peer groups, conflict resolution skills, good self-esteem, academic achievement and opportunities for participation in meaningful activities (WHO 2000b). These factors are closely aligned with the outcomes of *Every Child Matters* (Department for Education and Skills 2003).

The last decade has witnessed a growing interest in early prevention programmes to interrupt the developmental trajectories leading to poor outcomes for children and families. There is now a rapidly expanding evidence base showing that strategies to promote, prevent and intervene during childhood can offset the development of future problems and disorders in adolescence and adulthood. Our understanding of the epidemiological and social factors surrounding self-harm and suicide is becoming more sophisticated (Hawton 2005).

Suicide prevention

The prevention and control of suicide and self-harm is no easy task. However, high quality research suggests that it is feasibly possible, but involves a series of coordinated activities. WHO has suggested that these should focus on provision of the best possible conditions to bring up our children and youth, through the effective treatment of mental disorders, to the environmental control of risk factors (WHO 2000b).

Some European countries have defined suicide as a major public health concern and have developed suicide prevention centres that carry out research and inform health policy and planning. Suicide prevention centres are usually based in universities and carry out large multi-site studies.

One of the best known suicide prevention centres in the UK is the National Confidential Inquiry into Suicide and Homicide by People with Mental Illness (NCI/NCISH) based at the University of Manchester. This aims to reduce suicide rates by examining all deaths by suicide of people in contact with mental health services. Other key organisations are the Oxford Centre for Suicide Research where Keith Hawton and his team are based.

National strategies

A number of long-term strategies have been developed in the UK. Whilst most do not focus directly on self-harm, the majority address the issues and factors that often combine to cause young people to self-harm. Some of the overarching strategies apply to the UK, whereas others are country specific. In addition, some include specific plans for young people and high risk groups, such as Looked After Children.

England

The National Service Framework (NSF) for Children, Young People and Maternity Services is a ten-year programme that aims to bring about long-term and sustained improvements in children's health (Department of Health 2004). The NSF sets standards and defines service models for children across all NHS and social care settings. There are five core standards in the NSF which focus on involving children and families, interagency working, competent commissioning and care pathways. In addition, there are six specific standards which focus on children and young people with particular needs.

The National Service Framework for Children, Young People and Maternity Services

Standard 1: Promoting health and well-being, identifying needs and intervening early

Standard 2: Supporting parents

Standard 3: Child, young person and family centred services

Standard 4: Growing up into adulthood

Standard 5: Safeguarding and promoting the welfare of children and young people

Standard 6: Children and young people who are ill

Standard 7: Children in hospital

Standard 8: Disabled children and young people and those with complex needs

Standard 9: Mental health and psychological well-being of children and young people

Standard 10: Medicines for children and young people

Standard 11: Maternity services

The NSF does not address self-harm specifically, but most of the standards contain markers of good practice which health professionals should apply as part of their day-to-day practice with young people, parents and carers.

Standard 7: Children in hospital

This standard refers to the need for all staff to possess the skills to recognise and manage self-harm. It also states that all hospitals receiving and treating children and young people should have policies and liaison arrangements to deal with management of overdoses and self-harm, including self-mutilation and attempted suicide. The standard goes on to specify that staff should pay particular attention to ensuring proper medical and mental health care provision for self-harming and suicidal young people in A&E departments, where evidence suggests their needs can be badly neglected.

Standard 9: Mental health and psychological well-being of children and young people

This standard addresses mental health and psychological well-being of children and young people. This includes standards in relation to collaborative arrangements between multi-agency services (Department of Health 2004).

The need for health professionals to recognise self-harm and help identify support for young people is also stated in the government's strategy for children and young people's health, *Healthy Lives, Brighter Futures* (Department of Health 2009).

Suicide prevention

Reducing the mortality rate from suicide was identified as a key priority in the government's white paper, *Saving Lives: our healthier nation* (Department of Health 1999), which set out to reduce the death rate from suicide and undetermined injury by at least one-fifth by 2010. Action to help meet this target was later set out in the *National Suicide Prevention Strategy for England* (Department of Health 2002).

The Health Development Agency has published an evidence-based briefing on the effectiveness of preventative strategies for youth suicide and suicidal behaviour (NHS Health Development Agency 2002). This was published on behalf of the UK and Ireland Public Health Evidence Group and identifies all relevant systematic reviews, syntheses and meta-analyses relating to suicide by young people.

As part of Local Safeguarding Children Boards (LSCB), child death review panels are required to consider deaths of children and young people in each local area and identify lessons that can be learned to prevent future serious cases of self-harm and suicide (HM Government 2008).

Scotland

One in ten of the million children living in Scotland have mental health problems that interfere with their everyday lives. For many, this includes self-harm (Public Health Institute of Scotland 2003). Rates of suicide by people aged over 14 in Scotland have decreased by 12.5 per cent in the last decade (Samaritans 2008) (see Table 10.1).

Table 10.1 Number of deaths by suicide in 2006 (from Samaritans 2008)

Country	Number of deaths	Rates per 100,000 of people aged over 14
England	4191	10
Wales	300	12
Scotland	765	18
Northern Ireland	291	21
Republic of Ireland	409	12
UK total	5576	11
UK and RoI total	5985	9

Choose Life is a National programme which aims to improve the mental health and well-being of the Scottish population (Scottish Executive 2002). It includes a strategy and action plan to prevent suicide and provides joint multi-agency guidance relating to children and young people. The strategy forms a key part of the work of the National Programme for Improving Mental Health and Wellbeing in Scotland, which was launched in 2001. Among other priorities, this includes a target to reduce the suicide rate in Scotland by 20 per cent by 2013. Guidance issued as part of *Choose Life* seeks to raise awareness and defines the overarching roles and responsibilities of the relevant agencies supporting children and young people who self-harm. Three main priorities are identified as the following:

1   Supporting the improved coordination of efforts by local agencies to develop and implement local suicide prevention action plans.
2   Encouraging and supporting more innovative local voluntary services, community based and self-help initiatives that contribute to the prevention of suicide in local neighbourhoods and communities.
3   Developing and implementing local training programmes.

The Scottish Government has also published *Towards a Mentally Flourishing Scotland* which outlines six main priorities for health improvement, including the need to reduce the prevalence of suicide and self-harm.

Towards a Mentally Flourishing Scotland

1   Mentally healthy children, infants and young people
2   Mentally healthy later life
3   Mentally healthy communities
4   Mentally healthy employment and working life
5   Reducing the prevalence of suicide, self-harm and common mental health problems
6   Improving the quality of life of those experiencing mental health problems and mental illness

(Scottish Executive 2008)

Another promising initiative is *Building the Strengths Within*. This has been jointly published by the Scottish Development Centre for Mental Health and the Camelot Foundation, and aims to increase and share learning around young people from minority communities and self-harm (Scottish Development Centre for Mental Health and the Camelot Foundation 2005). The project is aimed at young people aged 16–25 from black and minority ethnic (BME) groups, including young refugees and asylum seekers, who self-harm or who are at risk of self-harm.

Talk to Me **action plan**

- To help people feel good about themselves
- To ensure early action is taken
- To respond to crises in people's lives
- To deal with the effects of suicide and self-harm
- To increase research and improve information
- To work with the media to ensure sensitive reporting on mental health and suicide
- To restrict access to things which could be used for suicide

Other Scottish public health initiatives have included *Breathing Space*, a helpline for young people with low mood or depression to offer advice and support and facilitate access to appropriate help and care services.

Wales

There are over half a million children living in Wales and they make up approximately one-fifth of the total population (Welsh Office 1997). Suicide rates of young people in Wales are higher than in England but lower than in Scotland or Northern Ireland (Welsh Assembly Government 2008) (see Table 10.1).

Talk to Me is the Welsh National action plan to reduce suicide and self-harm, and includes a particular focus on children and young people. The priority areas in the action plan are listed below (Welsh Assembly Government 2008).

Republic of Ireland

Suicide in Ireland rose dramatically in the 1990s and the increase was largely accounted for by young men (Cullen 2006). In the last decade however, the Republic of Ireland has seen the largest decrease in rates of suicide with a reduction of 14.5 per cent of deaths of people aged over 14 (Samaritans 2008) (see Table 10.1). Some have argued that this is partly due to the strong economic recovery experienced in Ireland from the prolonged slump of the 1980s to the boom of the 1990s.

Other factors that are thought to be important are the growth of multiculturalism and the reduced influence of the Catholic Church (Nolan *et al.* 2001). A report by Cullen (2006) on the coverage and treatment of suicide in the Irish print media stated that the prevention of suicide has not historically been given high priority in Ireland. Suicide prevention has received significantly smaller amounts of funding than road safety awareness, despite road traffic accidents accounting for fewer fatalities than deaths by suicide.

200 Preventing suicide and self-harm: a public health priority

The *Report of the National Task Force on Suicide* (Department of Health and Children 1998) helped set the policy context for suicide prevention. Although this does not focus specifically on children and adolescents, the report sets a framework to prevent suicide by young people. Following this report, the National Suicide Review Group formed and the National Office for Suicide Prevention was established as part of the Health Service Executive.

A number of key public health reports focusing on suicide prevention in Ireland have also been published. These include *Suicide in Ireland: Everyone's Problem* which highlighted a range of contributory factors (Bates 2005).

Northern Ireland

Over a quarter of Northern Ireland's population are children under the age of 18 (Northern Ireland Statistics and Research Agency 2002). However, very little robust epidemiological information about self-harm and suicidal behaviour among the child population is available. The widely cited research studies of 10,000 children published by the Office for National Statistics (Green *et al.* 2005) did not include children from the province.

The Health and Wellbeing Survey (Department of Health, Social Services and Public Safety 2001) looked at the Northern Ireland population in general. The survey concluded that people living in Northern Ireland are at greater risk of mental ill health than people in England and Scotland (Department of Health, Social Services and Public Safety 2001). This is partly due to higher levels of socio-economic deprivation, the ongoing civil troubles, and higher rates of mental health problems in adults (Northern Ireland Association for Mental Health and Sainsbury Centre for Mental Health 2004).

Prevention of suicide has been identified as a key area in Northern Ireland's strategy and action plan on Promoting Mental Health (Department of Health, Social Services and Public Safety 2003). In 2006, *Protect Life* was launched by the Department of Health, Social Services and Public Safety. This is Northern Ireland's five-year suicide prevention strategy and action plan until 2011. The strategy requires each Health and Social Services Board to develop a local *Protect Life* action plan which reflects the needs of children and young people.

Although rates of mental disorder across England, Wales and Scotland are thought to be broadly similar, Northern Ireland has the highest suicide rate in the UK with 21 per 100,000 young people over 14 years of age. This is an increase in 111 per cent since 1997 (Samaritans 2008) (see Table 10.1).

Prevention of self-harm

Interventions designed to reduce or eliminate self-harm have been researched, but this has mainly been with young adults. Fewer studies have been conducted with children and adolescents and we cannot rely with confidence upon extrapolation of findings with adults to support our work with young people (Livesey 2009).

In recent years there have been several major systematic reviews of universal or primary prevention programmes focused broadly on improving emotional health and psychological well-being (Harden *et al.* 2003; Wells *et al.* 2003; Edwards 2003). Several have included selective or indicated programmes addressing self-harm and suicide prevention.

What do we mean by prevention?

Prevention of self-harm involves universal or primary interventions which are aimed at the factors which contribute to self-harm and are focused on the health and well-being of children and young people in general. This includes the development of emotional resilience and healthy psychological coping strategies.

Secondary prevention is focused on reducing the prevalence of self-harm and involves early identification and interventions for young people at risk. This involves developing support systems in order that young people in distress can access help if they are struggling.

Tertiary prevention is concerned with providing support for those already struggling with self-harm and is often associated with harm minimisation. This can involve approaches to reduce repetition and harm minimisation strategies.

Healthy Lives, Brighter Futures, the Government's child health strategy highlights the need for the children's workforce to be able to recognise and identify support for young people who may be self-harming (Department of Health 2009).

Innovative approaches

Research on what works to prevent young people from self-harming is lacking. At the time of writing this book a large multi-centre trial has commenced and will run until 2016. The Self Harm Intervention Family Therapy (SHIFT) trial will involve around 800 young people, aged 11–17, and their families. It will be one of the largest and most comprehensive studies of its kind. Researchers will look at whether a whole-family approach, which focuses on the relationships, roles and communication patterns between family members, will enable families to work with young people to help them manage crises and emotional situations more effectively.

Participants in the SHIFT trial will have self-harmed more than once and will have required hospital admission for their injuries, although those diagnosed with severe depression or other serious mental disorders will not be asked to take part. The study is being funded by the National Institute for Health Research Health Technology Assessment programme and led by the University of Leeds and NHS Leeds. Sixteen other organisations will collaborate on the study by recruiting young people to the trial and delivering family therapy sessions in their local areas.

Projects such as the Manchester and Salford Self Harm Project aim to monitor patterns of self-harm across local populations, evaluate service effectiveness and provide local evidence on which service development and training strategies are based.

School and college based interventions

As many as one in five children and adolescents have mental health problems (Mental Health Foundation 1999; British Medical Association 2003) and up to one in ten children and young people aged 5–15 in England, Scotland and Wales will have a diagnosable mental disorder (Green *et al.* 2005).

This means that in an average secondary school with 1,000 pupils, as many as 50 will be depressed, between 10 and 20 will be anxious and between five and ten will have an eating disorder (YoungMinds 1999). This is clear evidence that children and young people are struggling, and many turn to self-harm in an attempt to cope.

Schools and colleges play a vital part in helping children develop emotional health and well-being and children and adolescents spend longer in school than any other environment (WHO 1997). One of the recommendations from the National Inquiry was that head teachers play a pivotal role in developing positive mental health strategies in schools, and that they should recognise the need to develop a whole school awareness of mental and emotional health issues.

Given that a large number of children and adolescents who self-harm are of school or college age there is huge potential to intervene in a positive way. Young people told the National Inquiry they feel it is important that counsellors rather than teachers should take on the role of supporting them with self-harm. In addition, the University of Oxford Centre for Suicide Research and the Samaritans recommend that schools should play a more prominent role, arguing that prevention needs to take place in the community and ideally within schools.

What can schools do?

A range of school-based professionals, including school nurses, educational psychologists, Special Educational Needs Coordinators (SENCOs), speech and language therapists, learning mentors, classroom support assistants, pastoral staff and school counsellors, play a key role in supporting pupils and students achieve their potential. Emotional health and well-being is now a core part of the national curriculum and personal, social and health education (PSHE) agenda.

School-based professionals, such as teachers and school nurses, are often the first to notice that a young person may be self-harming. They are in key positions to support young people and refer those who may require specialist assessment or treatment to specialist CAMHS or dedicated self-harm services.

> If there had been people to talk to at school then maybe I wouldn't have felt the need to start self-harming then.

Anti-bullying strategies and whole school approaches focused on emotional health and well-being appear to have a beneficial effect, but their outcomes in relation to self-harm are yet to be evaluated. Indeed, there is evidence that targeted interventions with individual young people at suicidal risk may be superior to whole school approaches or interventions at a group level (Thompson *et al.* 2000). In some areas of the country, ChildLine has been working with schools to set up the CHIPS (ChildLine in Partnership with Schools) Project. This helps schools set up schemes to encourage children and young people to support each other in school.

National strategies

Through the development of comprehensive programmes, universal approaches and targeted interventions, education service commissioners and professionals in schools are encouraged to focus on the development of emotional health and well-being in all areas of curriculum design and implementation.

There is presently a lack of evidence for curriculum-based universal suicide prevention programmes aimed at children and young people (NHS Health Development Agency 2002). As part of its public health programme, NICE has produced guidance in relation to social and emotional well-being in primary schools (NICE 2008). Although the guidelines omit to directly including self-harm, the suggested areas for investment by schools include problem solving, coping with stress, conflict resolution and understanding feelings. These are all areas of functioning which many young people who self-harm find difficult to manage on a day-to-day basis (McAuliffe *et al.* 2006).

The most important programmes that address mental health in schools have been the government-funded SEAL and TaMHS projects:

SEAL

The Social and Emotional Aspects of Learning (SEAL) programme (Department for Education and Skills 2005a) is part of the National Healthy Schools Programme (NHSP) (Department for Education and Skills 2005b). SEAL is a comprehensive approach to supporting the emotional and social skills that underpin effective learning and social and psychological well-being. The programme covers many areas that frequently challenge young people who self-harm, including making friends and getting on with others, bullying and managing changes.

In addition to curricular inputs to help support children to develop social problem solving skills and emotional processing skills as a means of preventing self-harm and suicidal thinking and behaviour, it is necessary to focus on whole school approaches to self-harm. For some children, school is part of the problem. Worries such as progress with work, assessments and peer relationships are very high indeed on children's lists of stressors (Morris 2008). Moreover, studies have suggested that there is a significant minority of pupils who do not feel that support is available in school, and who believe that relatively few teachers can be depended upon to offer timely or effective help when they are anxious, unhappy or worried on their own or others' behalf (Morris 2008).

TaMHS

The Targeted Mental Health in Schools (TaMHS) project is funded by the Department for Children, Schools and Families, and aims to transform the way in which children aged 5–13 can be supported to develop good mental health. The supporting materials include information on recognising and managing self-harm in schools. This draws on evidence-based advice for mental health professionals working with children and adolescents who self-harm (Wolpert *et al.* 2006). Importantly, the evidence suggests that whilst school-based interventions can improve knowledge and attitudes towards self-harm among young people, they have not been shown to increase help seeking behaviour among high risk groups such as young men and those who have already self-harmed (Wolpert *et al.* 2006).

Training and support for schools

Despite government policy to improve child mental health training for frontline professionals (Department of Health 2004), and the very high level of contact teachers have with children and young people who self-harm, training about self-harm and mental health problems in general for teachers and other school-based staff has been lacking (Gowers *et al.* 2004).

Furthermore, when faced with students who self-harm, teachers and other school and college staff often need the support of specialist mental health services. In fulfilling their responsibilities to support the promotion of mental health and by responding appropriately to suicidal or self-harming pupils, schools can draw on expertise from external services and agencies in the form of consultation and advisory support (Morris 2008). In addition, since many young people who self-harm turn to their friends for support, there is a need to address school based peer support schemes and systems, such as student mentors who are trained to support other students who are having problems.

Stigma

There is growing acknowledgement that stigma is a major problem experienced by many people with mental health problems and people who self-harm. The impact of stigma has been recognised since Erving Goffman (1963) published a book subtitled *Notes on the Management of Spoiled Identity*. In this book he traced the origins of stigma back to ancient Greece where a brand or visible mark was placed on the foreheads of people in 'tainted' groups, such as traitors, or to identify an animal or slave. However, it has only been in recent years that public campaigns have begun to promote better understanding about mental health and challenging stigma.

See Beyond the Label

YoungMinds have published *See Beyond the Label*, which is a comprehensive training manual to help professionals develop effective support services for young people who self-harm. It provides opportunities to think about our attitudes towards self-harm, and to increase our understanding of why children and young people harm themselves. Based on feedback from young people, the resource reminds professionals that:

- young people rarely ask for help directly
- they often choose to talk to a friend rather than parents or professionals
- they do not want adults to overreact
- they do not want to be called self-harmers.

YoungMinds also encourages professionals and school staff to seek out ways to tackle the stigma commonly associated with expressions of mental distress, and to ensure the involvement of young people who self-harm in the design, implementation and evaluation of local self-harm protocols (YoungMinds 2006). There are four key aims underpinning the training:

- provide opportunities for all of us to think about our attitudes to self-harm;
- increase our understanding about why children and young people self-harm;
- seek out ways to tackle the stigma commonly associated with expressions of mental distress; and
- ensure the involvement of young people who self-harm in the design, implementation and evaluation of local self-harm protocols.

Stigma and families

It is not only the young person who is affected by stigma. Often the parents, siblings and friends of a young person who self-harms also frequently suffer as a result of negative attitudes and behaviours. Parents may be unsure whether to tell family and friends about their child's self-harm, or keep it secret. Just as stress can build up in a young person who has no appropriate source of support, so too can parents and carers struggle when there is no available network of support.

The *Time to Change* campaign in the UK aims to end mental health discrimination through various events and films, though it does not focus particularly on young people or self-harm. *Time to Change* is enlisting the help of celebrities and people known to the public, who are willing to speak out about their own experiences of mental health and illness (www.time-to-change.org.uk/home).

As well as UK stigma campaigns, some of the individual countries have embarked on activities to eliminate stigma. Using TV, radio and bus shelter advertisements *See Me* has been launched across Scotland and calls for greater awareness and understanding of self-harm among Scotland's many different cultures. In particular, the campaign aims to tackle the issue of self-harm amongst black and minority ethnic communities (www.seemescotland.org.uk). Produced as part of *See Me, Just Like Me* uses animation and cartoons to help children and young people learn about the effects of stigma and how to tackle it. The *Just Like Me* website includes stories about young people who self-harm (www.justlikeme.org.uk).

In addition, the national charity Rethink has been running an anti-stigma campaign in Northern Ireland since 2007. This has featured TV, outdoor and bus advertising, and a number of service users have trained as media volunteers and shared their stories and experiences with the local and national media.

Tackling stigma framework

A model of intervention for tackling stigma in children, young people and their families has been developed by Gale (2007). This can be implemented within CAMHS and children's services in general (see Figure 10.1).

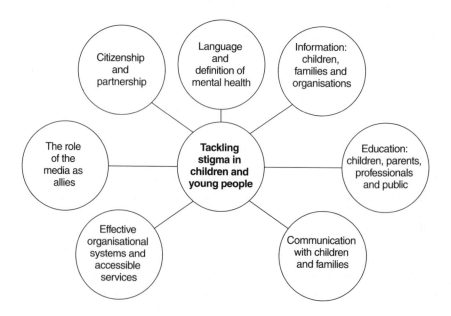

Figure 10.1 Tackling stigma framework (Gale 2007)

Media, social networking and self-harm

Against the context of individual factors we have discussed, children and young people are living in a society where there is a high expectation of instant gratification and quick fixes. Young people are growing up in a culture where people do not expect to have to wait to have their wishes and needs fulfilled. From material goods, such as houses, holidays, clothes and music, there is increased instant access through loans and 24-hour facilities, to communications with email, MSN, social websites and mobile phones.

Today's young people have a world of technology at their fingertips. Adolescents use the internet for the purpose of socialising and communicating with others more than any other age group (Lenhart *et al.* 2001; Gross 2004). Like many closeted or stigmatised behaviours, self-harm communities and outlets flourish on the world wide web (Norris *et al.* 2006; Biddle *et al.* 2008).

Perhaps the best known examples of this are the 'Pro Ana' and 'Pro Mia', websites which respectively promote anorexia nervosa and bulimia nervosa as lifestyle choices rather than eating disorders. The internet may appeal particularly to young people who are shy, socially anxious or isolated, or those who feel marginalised (Subrahmanyam *et al.* 2004). This is because it provides a relatively low risk venue for finding others who share their perceived or real differences (McKenna and Green 2002). Young people who self-harm are one such group. Mobile phones, emails, instant messaging and social networking sites can be hugely influential in both preventing and promoting self-harm.

When we consider that many young people who self-harm are reluctant to confide in adults and are three times more likely to turn to a friend than a professional (Mental Health Foundation and Camelot Foundation 2006), social networking is something of an untapped resource. However, it is important that young people should not be in a position where they receive confidences about self-harm without effective support systems being in place (Fortune *et al.* 2005). As children turn to their friends for advice, they need help not only coping with their own emotional problems, but also in supporting friends who may be in distress. The establishment of peer support, 'buddy schemes' and mentoring systems in schools have been a helpful step in this regard (Morris 2008).

Are self-harm websites helpful or harmful?

Evidence has shown that young adults who self-harm often use websites to gain empathy and understanding, a sense of community and ways of coping with social and psychological distress. This, in turn, leaves them feeling better understood and less isolated (Baker and Fortune 2008). These benefits, as well as possible risks, associated with such websites need to be understood further as they are increasingly used by children and young people.

In their discussions with professionals, young people who self-harm describe two different types of website. First are those run by professionals, and second are those created by people who self-harm. The anonymity of not having face-to-face contact can encourage youngsters to be fairly explicit about their self-harm, which can have a negative effect on vulnerable young people who may be tempted to imitate behaviours. Often, these discussions take place far from the scrutiny of parents or carers.

The boundaries of cyber relationships are at the discretion of the young people who may not have reached a level of maturity whereby they can impose their own limits on unhealthy relationships. Furthermore issues such as bullying can be rife, as was the case with so-called 'happy slapping' through text messaging, which was reported a few years ago on national television. The National Inquiry recommends that reputable sites are publicised more widely to young people to ensure that they can access the most appropriate advice. The role of the media in promoting positive attitudes towards self-harm and suicide has been discussed earlier in the book.

An interesting study by Whitlock and colleagues explored the use of the internet as a coping strategy for young people who self-harm (Whitlock *et al.* 2006). They used observational data from blogs and message boards to investigate how adolescents solicit and share information about self-harm. Findings showed that online access clearly provided essential social support for otherwise isolated adolescents, but the authors concluded that it may also normalise and encourage self-harm and add potentially lethal behaviours to the repertoire of young people who are already self-harming and those exploring alternative coping strategies (Whitlock *et al.* 2006).

Instant messaging

The needs and intentions of young people who self-harm are often communicated by mobile phone. The growth and availability of mobile phone technology has changed the landscape in which young people communicate and receive support from family and friends. The large majority of young people own a mobile phone, and most keep them on their person at all times. Conversations with young people in general suggest that many could not contemplate the idea of switching off their phones and being unavailable, even during the night.

For those that self-harm, texts and emails are often a critical communication or cry for help. For those that receive them, the communications may indicate that their distressed friend is in need of support. Some have argued that we are at risk of creating a culture whereby young people feel increasingly less able to wait, to contain their own feelings, and to go some way towards sorting problems out themselves before calling upon the support of others. PAPYRUS has published guidance for parents and carers to support their children to take a safe and responsible approach to the cyber world, or who may have concerns that their child is depressed or suicidal (PAPYRUS 2008).

Modernising e-access to services

It is concerning that for some young people who self-harm there is a paradox. In this era of increased technological communication they find themselves more isolated and less likely to discuss their difficulties face-to-face. A recent report by YouthNet highlights how important modern technology is for young people. They found that 82 per cent of young people used the internet at some point to look for information and advice, and use a range of different mediums to access this. This provides a key opportunity to provide services differently and in a way that children and young people find helpful.

Several charities, including the Samaritans, have attempted to respond to this by providing 'electronic befriending', using the internet to enable young people to directly access support services. Some UK CAMHS teams have attempted to adapt their communications to meet the needs of young people in the twenty-first century. By using text, email and instant messaging they have attempted to improve access and engagement. However, this is not widespread and the effectiveness of this change in communication strategy is yet to be evaluated.

Self-harm and suicide training packages

With appropriate training, health professionals and others can become skilled in early and accurate identification of self-harm and suicidal risk (Horowitz *et al.* 2001). There are several training packages available to help professionals become more knowledgeable and skilled in assessing and working with young people who self-harm. Two examples are ASIST and STORM.

ASIST

Applied Suicide Intervention Skills Training (ASIST) is a suicide 'first aid' training programme developed in Canada. It is suitable for professionals and lay people and consists of a two-day interactive package on suicide risk management. The aim of ASIST is to prepare caregivers to recognise suicide risk factors, and develop skills to intervene during crisis. The programme addresses attitudes to self-harm and explores the resources available within local communities. ASIST has been successfully implemented in a number of countries worldwide. It is recognised by the Department of Health in England and has been adopted as a national suicide intervention training programme by the Scottish Executive Government.

STORM

Skills Based Training on Risk Management (STORM) is a suicide prevention training package which can be used as part of an overall suicide prevention strategy by organisations in statutory and voluntary sectors. It can be delivered either in a short modular format or over one or two days. The package covers assessment, crisis management, crisis prevention and problem solving when working with potentially suicidal service users. A version for children and young people is available in addition to the adult format. Facilitators are professionals, non-professionals or service users with relevant experience who have been trained to deliver the package in a cascade model.

Summary

A reduction in suicidal behaviour, both fatal and non-fatal, is part of the *Health for all Targets* of the World Health Organization. However, there is a serious lack of information about which treatments or preventative strategies are effective for young people who self-harm (WHO 1997). Knowledge regarding prevention is limited. Furthermore, there has been relatively little empirical work on the treatment of adolescent suicides. Further research is required to identify the long-term costs of self-harm by young people and to inform strategic policy and planning decisions.

Campaigns to promote awareness, recognition and understanding about self-harm are crucial if the helping and caring professions and wider public are to improve outcomes for young people who self-harm (McDougall and Brophy 2006). Many young people who self-harm experience rejection, abuse and trauma, and encounter stigma when seeking help for their self-harm. This is unacceptable in modern caring and support services.

Innovative approaches to prevention and intervention should be developed across organisations, services and professional groups who work with children and young people. Improving ways to engage young people through creative arts, media and social networking are a few ways in which professionals can help make a difference.

11 Self-harm and the legal framework

Key points:

- It is important that professionals helping children and young people who self-harm are clear about the legal frameworks within which they work. Regardless of the context in which they practice, professionals should be familiar with human rights legislation, children's rights and mental health law and how these frameworks interact.
- Like any child or young person, those who self-harm have a right to privacy, dignity and respect. Despite these principles, young people often report that they are not involved in decisions, frequently have their privacy, dignity and confidentiality compromised and do not feel that professionals respect them.
- Children have a right to protection from all forms of violence. Professionals and the organisations within which they work must protect children from all forms of physical and mental violence, injury or abuse and neglect, including protecting children from suicide and self-harm.
- Evaluating competency is an essential part of the assessment process prior to the provision of any assessment or treatment for self-harm by a child or young person. Children's competence is determined by their maturity and understanding rather than their fixed chronological age. This means that they may be competent to make one treatment decision but not another.
- Children's and young people's rights to confidentiality should be strictly observed. Health professionals should have a clear understanding of their duties of confidentiality, and any limits to such an obligation should be made clear to the child or young person who has the capacity to understand.
- Professionals may be concerned that sharing information about a young person's suicidal self-harming behaviour may breach their right to confidentiality. This is often the case when working with teenagers where the views of the young person and their parents are important. Whilst it is vital to have a working knowledge of the legal frameworks involved, simply asking the young person and parents about these issues can often be helpful and need not involve any breach of confidentiality.

Introduction

Care and treatment decisions affecting children and young people can often be complex, and it is essential that health professionals understand the different statutory frameworks within which they work. During the last few years there have been several changes to the law affecting children and young people. There have been amendments to the Children Act 1989 and the Mental Health Act 1983, and the main provisions in the Mental Capacity Act 2005 apply to 16- and 17-year-olds. There have also been amendments to the Domestic Violence, Crime and Victims Act 2004.

It is crucially important that changes to the law affecting the care and treatment of children and adolescents who are suicidal or self-harming are understood by health professionals and other adults who work with these young people.

This chapter is intended to provide guidance to health professionals about legal issues affecting the care and treatment of young people who self-harm. It clarifies the law, and offers practical guidance on dealing with common difficulties that arise on a day-to-day basis. These include dilemmas related to confidentiality, consent and refusal. For the purpose of this chapter, the term treatment refers to paediatric, psychiatric, psychological and psychotherapeutic interventions. It is necessary for readers to consider the range of issues set out in this chapter in order to understand how the various legal frameworks combine.

Some professionals, such as nurses and doctors, have responsibilities that are enshrined within their duties of care and codes of professional practice. All are required to ensure that children and young people are kept safe. Health professionals practise in a culture of litigation and their duty to care must be brokered with a wider responsibility to enable children to reach their fullest potential (Department for Education and Skills 2003).

Human rights and young people

Professionals who work with children in any context should be familiar with human rights legislation. The European Convention on Human Rights, the United Nations Convention on the Rights of the Child and the Human Rights Act 1998 provide the overarching human rights framework.

The European Convention on Human Rights (ECHR)

The ECHR was passed by the Council of Europe in 1950 and came into force in 1953. It was intended to give binding effect to the guarantee of various rights and freedoms contained in the UN Declaration on Human Rights, adopted several years earlier.

United Nations Convention on the Rights of the Child (UNCRC)

The UNCRC is the first legally binding international instrument to incorporate the full range of human rights. In 1989 world leaders decided that children needed a special convention because people under 18 years often need special care and protection. The leaders also wanted to make sure that the world recognised that children have human rights too (Harbour 2008).

The UNCRC establishes a range of civil, political, socio-economic and cultural rights that apply to all children and young people. As well as several important articles, there are two guiding principles that professionals who work with children and young people must always take into account in their day-to-day work:

1 There is a need to consider the best interests and views of the child.
2 Decisions in relation to children and young people must be made in a manner consistent with their evolving capacities. This means that as children mature and grow up towards independence, their views and wishes should be given greater weight in the decision making process.

Article 19 of the UNCRC entitles children to the right to protection from all forms of violence. States must take measures to protect children from all formals of physical and mental violence, injury or abuse and neglect. This includes a requirement to take measures to protect children from suicide and serious self-harm. This is therefore important when considering harm minimisation strategies which were discussed earlier in the book.

The Human Rights Act

The Human Rights Act (HRA) was passed in 1998 and became operational in 2000. It incorporates the rights enshrined in the European Convention on Human Rights into UK domestic law. This requires public authorities, organisations and professionals to take into account human rights in their day-to-day work with children and young people. The following articles are included in the HRA, of which article 1 is the convention. Article 2 dictates that authorities have a positive obligation to protect life.

Human rights law has lead to an increasing recognition that children and young people have rights and entitlements and can often make decisions for themselves.

Human Rights (articles)

1 Right to life
2 Protection from torture and inhuman or degrading treatment or punishment
3 Protection from slavery and forced labour

4 Right to liberty and security
5 Right to a fair trial
6 Protection from retrospective criminal offences
7 Protection of private and family life
8 Freedom of thought, conscience and religion
9 Freedom of expression
10 Freedom of assembly and association
11 Right to marry and found a family
12 Freedom from discrimination

Children's rights

The Children Act 1989 is a key legal framework governing the care and welfare of all children and young people under 18. Whilst the Children Act has been amended since it first came into force, most importantly by the Adoption and Children Act 2002 and the Children Act 2004, the original Act remains intact and in use today. The Children Act brings together private and public law provisions in a single legislative framework for law affecting children. It attempts to strike a balance between the rights of children, the responsibilities of both parents to their child and the duty of the state to intervene when the child's welfare requires it (Department for Children, Schools and Families 2008).

Respecting rights

As children and young people get older and move towards independence, their involvement in decision making increases. Whatever the age of the child, it is always important to keep them as fully informed and involved as possible. They should receive clear and detailed information in a format that is appropriate to their age and developmental understanding.

Like any child or young person, those who self-harm have a right to privacy, dignity and respect. Despite these principles, many of which are enshrined in human rights law, young people often report that they are not involved in decisions, frequently have their privacy, dignity and confidentiality compromised and do not feel that professionals respect them. This is unacceptable, and professionals must improve their practice in this area. Some young people feel they are not made aware of their rights:

> There needs to be more awareness of our choices – of not having a parent there with you if that is what we want.
>
> Casey, 16

Competence, capacity and consent

The United Nations Convention on the Rights of the Child and the Children Act (1989) entitles children to participatory decision making rights. Health service professionals are therefore obliged to give children and young people any information necessary to ensure their full participation in decision making. However, it is important to state that this does not necessarily mean children make the final decision, and this right may be mediated through the law on consent (Lansdown 2000).

When working with children and young people who self-harm, health professionals are frequently required to consider consent issues. For example, they may be faced with a child who refuses to enter an ambulance to attend hospital after an overdose. Alternatively, they may be asked by an adolescent not to share information with parents about cutting.

Making appropriate care and treatment decisions is not always straightforward, and professionals and other colleagues may sometimes disagree or make poorly informed choices. Young people have said clarity about confidentiality and consent is important to them (Mental Health Foundation and Camelot Foundation 2006), and it is important that health professionals carefully consider the legal implications of any decision they take.

Competence and capacity

Evaluating competency and capacity is an essential part of the assessment process prior to the provision of any assessment or treatment for self-harm by a child or young person. Children's competence is determined by their maturity and understanding rather than their fixed chronological age. This means that they may be competent to make one treatment decision but not another.

A person with the capacity to consent should be able to:

- understand in broad terms what the treatment is, what it is for and why it is being proposed;
- understand the principle benefits, risks and alternatives to the treatment being proposed;
- understand the likely consequences of not receiving the treatment being proposed;
- retain the above information for long enough to make an informed decision; and
- make a choice that is free from external pressure an secondary gain.

Consent by children under 16

Consent to medical treatment by or for children can be complex and requires a balance between preserving the principle of legal autonomy for children, whilst providing protection to safeguard their physical and mental health.

Within the framework of UK law, children and young people can do different things at different ages (Whotton 2002). Children under 16 can consent to treatment if they are deemed to be competent to do so. In order for consent to be valid, the child or young person must be capable of consenting, the consent must be freely given and the child or young person involved must be given appropriate information.

Gillick competence

In 1980, what was then the Department of Health and Social Security (DHSS), issued guidance on family planning services. The guidance suggested that in certain situations, a physician could lawfully prescribe contraception for a girl under 16 without the consent of her parents.

Five years later in 1985, the DHSS guidance was challenged in court by Victoria Gillick, the mother of five girls all aged under 16. Judge Scarman, who heard the case, concluded that 'the parental right to determine whether or not their minor child below the age of 16 will have medical treatment terminates if and when the child achieves sufficient understanding and intelligence to enable him or her to understand fully what is proposed'. This became known popularly as the test of 'Gillick competence', and the effect was to allow a competent child under the age of 16 a right to consent to treatment without the necessity to obtain parental consent (Harbour 2008).

Also ruling on the Gillick case, Lord Fraser set out guidelines to help determine competence, but in straightforward terms, this requires a child under 16 who has sufficient understanding and intelligence to enable him or her to fully understand what is being proposed (NSPCC 2008b). This is commonly referred to as the 'Fraser ruling'.

However, competence may vary according to the decision being proposed. A child or young person may be competent to make one decision but not another. Therefore, any assessment of a child or young person's capacity to consent must be 'decision specific'. To illustrate, consent for one thing (such as the assessment of self-harm) does not necessarily mean consent for another thing (such as referral for psychological treatment for self-harm). Competence may also fluctuate, particularly when there is mental disorder, and therefore consent for treatment decisions must always be kept under review.

Consent by young people aged 16 and 17

The assessment of capacity and of the ability to make decisions and consent to treatment is different for young people aged 16 and 17. The Mental Capacity Act 2005 provides that all people over 16 have the right to autonomy and independent decision making unless it can be shown that they lack capacity as defined in the Mental Capacity Act. Where young people lack capacity, decisions can be taken on their behalf in accordance with the legal provisions set out in the Act.

Treatment without consent

Care and treatment can be provided to children and young people without their consent in certain situations. This is where they lack capacity, and life saving treatment or treatment to prevent serious harm can be provided within the common law. There are also circumstances when the Mental Health Act 1983 can be used to provide physical treatment against a young person's wishes.

Research has shown that children who are given life saving treatment for severe eating disorders without their consent have been later grateful for treatment (Faith 2002). It has been suggested that suicidal children and young people may be similarly appreciative (Leighton 2007).

Mental Capacity Act – assessing capacity

Excepting situations when the Mental Health Act applies, the concept of mental capacity is central to decisions about treatment for a child or young person who refuses it. The Mental Capacity Act (MCA) 2005 provides the legal framework for adults who lack capacity to make decisions themselves. The Act does not generally apply to children aged under 16. However, there are two exceptions to this:

- The Court of Protection can make decisions about a child's property or finances if the child lacks capacity to make such decisions and is likely to still lack capacity to make financial decisions when they reach the age of 18.
- Offences of ill treatment or wilful neglect of a person who lacks capacity can also apply to victims younger than 16.

The main provisions of the MCA apply to 16- and 17-year-olds. There are several guiding principles enshrined in the Act:

- A person must be assumed to have capacity unless it is established that they lack capacity.
- A person is not to be treated as unable to make a decision unless all practicable steps to help them do so have been taken without success.
- A person is not to be treated as unable to make a decision merely because they are likely to make an unwise decision.
- An act done or decision made using the Act must be done or made in the person's best interests.

Having capacity to make a decision means having the ability to understand information, weigh up this information and come to an informed decision. People are said to lack capacity if they cannot do one or more of the following four things:

- understand information that is given to them
- retain information for long enough to able to make the decision
- use the information to make the decision
- verbally or non-verbally communicate their decision.

People carrying out acts in connection with the care and treatment of a young person aged 16 or 17 who lacks capacity to consent, will generally have protection from liability, as long as the person carrying out the act has taken all reasonable steps to establish that the young person lacks capacity (National Institute for Mental Health in England 2009).

When assessing the young person's best interests, the person providing care or treatment must consult those involved in the young person's care and anyone else interested in their welfare, which may include parents. Care should be taken not to unlawfully breach the young person's right to confidentiality. In the event that there are disagreements about the care, treatment or welfare of a young person aged 16 or 17 who lacks capacity, the case may be heard in the family courts or the Court of Protection.

Mental health legislation

The Mental Health Act (MHA) 1983 is concerned primarily with the circumstances in which people with mental disorders can be detained for assessment or treatment without consent. Most provisions apply to people of all ages, but there are additional safeguards for the care and treatment of children and young people.

Professionals who work with children and young people need to have a working knowledge of the MHA 1983 which was amended in 2007 to make nine key changes all applicable to children and young people (see Table 11.1).

Table 11.1 The nine key changes to the Mental Health Act

Key change	
1	A simplified single definition of mental disorder
2	Abolished the treatability test and introduced an Appropriate Medical Treatment Test
3	Requirement that age-appropriate services are available to any patients admitted to hospital who are aged under 18
4	Broadening of the professional groups that can take particular roles
5	Right for patients to apply to court to displace their nearest relative
6	Access to advocacy when under compulsion
7	New safeguards for patients receiving ECT
8	Supervised Community Treatment to allow a patient detained on a treatment order to receive their treatment in the community
9	Referral to a Tribunal where patients do not apply themselves

The MHA 2007 introduced five guiding principles through a revised Code of Practice (COP). These are intended to help professionals apply the Mental Health Act and Code of Practice in particular situations. The guiding principles are:

* purpose
* least restriction
* respect
* participation
* effectiveness, efficiency and equity.

Professionals must have regard to, and follow, the advice contained in the COP or be able to justify why they are not able to do so.

Chapter 36 of the COP is concerned with children and young people. As well as the guiding principles, it contains some key factors to acknowledge when considering use of the Act. These include the welfare principle, consideration of the principle of 'best interests' and the need to involve children and young people in treatment decisions.

What are the particular changes that affect children and young people?

The main amendments that affect children and young people refer to age-appropriate services; consent to treatment which was discussed earlier; and electro-convulsive therapy.

Age-appropriate facilities

The National Service Framework for Children, Young People and Maternity Services sets the expectation that young people admitted to hospital for mental health treatment should have access to appropriate care in an environment suited to their age and development (Department of Health 2004).

Section 31 of the Mental Health Act 2007 amends the Mental Health Act 1983 to place a duty on hospital managers to ensure that patients under 18 who are admitted to hospital for mental disorder are accommodated in an environment that is suitable for their age (subject to their needs). This is set out in section 131A of the Mental Health Act 1983 and the provision applies to both informal and detained patients. An age-appropriate environment refers not just to the physical layout, but to the accommodation, staff and facilities that children and young people need to fulfil their personal, educational and social development whilst in hospital (McDougall *et al.* 2009).

For all children under 16, and most young people aged 16 or 17 who require an inpatient mental health service, the most appropriate environment will be within a child and adolescent inpatient service. However, young people aged 16 or 17 may be admitted to adult mental health wards if this is the most suitable environment to meet their needs. In the exceptional case where a young person cannot be accommodated in a dedicated child or adolescent ward, discrete accommodation within an adult mental health ward is permissible if appropriate CAMHS support, robust safeguarding measures and age-appropriate facilities are made available. In determining whether the environment is suitable, hospital managers must consult a person with experience in child and adolescent mental health.

Zone of parental control

Whilst not part of statute, the concept of the 'zone of parental control' (ZPC) was introduced by the updated Mental Health Act Code of Practice. This states that in certain circumstances, parents can consent on behalf of their child if a decision is said to fall within the ZPC.

There are no clear rules on what may fall within the ZPC, and each decision needs to be considered in the light of the particular circumstances at the time. Factors such as the potential impact that the decision will have on the child or young person, their age and maturity, the nature of the treatment being considered and whether the child or young person is objecting to the treatment should all be considered before it can be decided whether the decision falls inside or outside the zone.

In assisting professionals to determine whether a decision falls within the ZPC, the COP sets out the following guidelines:

- Is this a decision that a parent would usually be expected to make, having regard to what is considered to be within the realms of normal parenting and human rights?
- Are there any indicators that the parent might not act in the best interests of their child or young person?

The less confident the professional that the answer to these questions is 'yes', the more likely it will be that the decision in question falls outside the zone of parental control.

It may be appropriate to involve a court to intervene where parents refuse to consent for treatment (considered by a physician to be necessary) to be given to their child; or where there are child protection concerns that impact negatively on parental ability to act in the best interests of their child.

Refusal and emergency treatment for self-harm

The Children Act 1989 refers to circumstances where a child can refuse to be assessed, examined or treated. The provisions state that, not withstanding any court direction, a child with sufficient understanding to make an informed treatment decision can refuse to be assessed, examined or treated. However, as we will see later, parents can sometimes consent on their child's behalf.

However, in rare circumstances, the court can override such a refusal if it is deemed to compromise the best interests of the child. There are several circumstances where the refusal by a young person of potentially life saving treatment could be overruled. They might not fully comprehend the conse- quences of his or her decision, they may be acting under the undue influence of another, their emotional distress may impair their judgement, or the young person's behaviour shows that they are deeply ambivalent about the decision, for example by initially seeking help from emergency services (NICE 2004a).

Practitioners can also use the common law to treat a child or young person without their consent in a life threatening emergency. This is when immedi- ate action is needed to either save a life or protect them from serious further harm. In such cases, the treatment must be reasonable and limited to what- ever appears necessary to resolve the emergency. The courts have stated that doubt should be resolved in favour of the preservation of life, and it is accept- able to undertake treatment to preserve life or prevent irreversible serious deterioration of the patient's condition. Emergency treatment for self-harm only applies to physical interventions for self-harm, such as resuscitation after a cardiac arrest induced by a serious overdose or life saving surgery after self- injurious behaviour.

Confidentiality and information sharing

The purpose of sharing information is to ensure young people who harm themselves or are perceived to be at risk of self-harm, as well as suicide, are given the help and support they need. A commitment to sharing information and the need for clear communication across agencies is crucial if young peo- ple are at serious risk from self-harm or suicide attempts. However, this needs to be balanced against the rights of young people to confidentiality which can only be breached in certain circumstances.

The right to confidentiality applies to children and young people. Where they are able to make decisions about the use and disclosure of information they have given in confidence, the views of children and young people should be respected in the same way that those of adults are respected (National Institute for Mental Health in England 2009).

Can confidentiality be breached?

A child or young person's right to confidentiality can be limited in certain circumstances but this should only be on a 'need to know basis'. This is where a risk of serious harm or abuse is suspected and safeguarding concerns justify disclosure without consent (Department for Skills and Education 2006a).

For example, if a health professional is concerned that a child or young person is going to kill themselves, information relating to this risk can be disclosed without consent, even if the young person is competent. It is important to remember that any decisions concerning the disclosure of information about a child or young person without their consent must always be proportionate to protect the needs in question (Department for Skills and Education 2006b).

Guidance from the Department of Health on confidentiality for health professionals is available, and staff working for the NHS are obliged to follow the NHS Code of Practice on Confidentiality (Department of Health 2003b).

What do young people think about confidentiality?

Quite understandably, young people are often reluctant to disclose their self-harm due to fears that their right to confidentiality might be compromised (NSPCC 2009). The CASE study sent questionnaires to 30,000 young people aged 15 or 16. Reassured that their confidentiality would be protected and that answers would be anonymised, 70 per cent admitted to self-harming at some stage during their adolescence (Madge *et al.* 2008).

This appears to confirm that confidentiality is important to young people who self-harm. The CASE study finding has previously been supported in a qualitative research study by Le Surf and Lynch (1999). Investigators set out to understand the perceptions and attitudes of young people towards counselling. The need for confidentiality was highlighted as a consistent theme. This was often associated with stigma and the effects of having counselling, as well as a deeper experience of shamefulness.

Research and surveys of service user views confirm that young people may often not want others to know they are having counselling for their self-harm. For many, their history, background and personal information has been shared among many professionals, and often the child or young person is unaware of who knows what about them. They frequently have an overwhelming sense that their privacy and boundaries are being invaded (Edwards 2007). It is therefore crucially important to be clear about the limits of confidentiality and the circumstances within which disclosure to a third party would be necessary.

As guidance for public health practitioners issued by the NSPCC points out, these issues mean that strict reporting requirements have to be balanced against young people's wishes and their well-being (NSPCC 2009). This generates a range of moral, ethical and legal issues for professionals who work with young people who self-harm, each of which needs to be fully considered. For example, if a young person insists that their parents are not informed about their self-harm, and they may be at significant risk of harm, health professionals are faced with a potentially difficult decision. In making an informed decision we should consider at least three issues:

1   *What are my moral and ethical obligations?*
     What do I believe is the right thing to do or not to do?

2   *What are my contractual obligations?*
    What does my employer require me to do or not to do?

3   *What are the legal obligations?*
    What does the law require me to do or not to do?

Professional concerns about confidentiality

It is not only children and young people that have concerns about confidentiality and the use and disclosure of information. So too do professionals who may be concerned that sharing information may breach a young person's right to confidentiality. This is often the case when working with teenagers where the views of the young person and their parents are important.

However, whilst it is important to have a working knowledge of the legal frameworks, simply asking the young person and parents about these issues can often be helpful and need not involve any breach of confidentiality. This is providing that the person requesting or providing the information does not reveal any personal confidential information that the parent or carer would not legitimately know anyway (National Institute for Mental Health in England 2009).

Parental responsibility and involvement

Parental responsibility is defined in the Children Act 1989 as 'all the rights, duties, powers, responsibilities and authority which by law a parent has in relation to a child and his property'. Wherever the care and treatment of a child who has self-harmed is being considered, the person, or persons, with parental responsibility must be identified, and their views sought as appropriate.

Who has parental responsibility?

The person with parental responsibility is usually, but not always, the child or young person's parent. However, it is important to establish who has parental responsibility and whether this is shared with another parent or the local authority.

First, this is important because the person or persons with responsibility may be able to consent to their child's treatment. This may involve authorising admission to hospital for treatment of self-harm. Second, children's legislation determines that it is good practice to involve those with parental responsibility even if they do not consent to their child's treatment.

The mother of a child will automatically have parental responsibility for her child unless the child has been adopted by someone else. The father has responsibility for his child if he either:

*   was married to the child's mother at the time of the child's birth
*   acquires parental responsibility by becoming registered on the birth certificate

- makes a parental responsibility agreement with the child's mother
- acquires parental responsibility through a court order.

Step-parents may acquire parental responsibility through a residence order, by adopting the child or becoming their legal guardian as defined in the Children Act.

The local authority can also acquire parental responsibility for a child. This is through a care order and, with restrictions, under an emergency protection order. However, the local authority does not acquire parental responsibilities if a child is voluntarily accommodated by the local authority (National Institute for Mental Health in England 2009).

Shared parental responsibility

Where more than one person has parental responsibility for a child, each may act alone, without the other, in meeting that responsibility. This means that, for example, professionals can lawfully provide treatment to the child with the authority of one parent, even though both parents have parental responsibility.

A person who does not have parental responsibility for a child but has care of the child may do what is reasonable under the circumstances to safeguard or promote the child's welfare. Whether or not the intervention can be considered reasonable depends on the urgency or seriousness of the situation and the extent to which it is practicable to consult a person with parental responsibility (National Institute for Mental Health in England 2009). This allows professionals to act in emergencies where treatment following self-harm is considered necessary.

Summary

The law in relation to children and young people who self-harm is complex. Health professionals should have easy access to legal advice and consultation to ensure their practice is lawful. All professionals who work with children and young people should be clear about their professional obligations and the various legal frameworks affecting the care and treatment of young people. The National Institute for Mental Health in England (2009) has published a guide for professionals on the legal aspects of the care and treatment of children and young people with mental disorder. This is helpful in assisting health professionals to navigate the complex legal terrain within which they work with young people who are suicidal or self-harming.

Issues of confidentiality should be openly discussed with the young person and jointly understood. Where confidentiality needs to be compromised in relation to risk, it should be done respectfully and openly. Normally, a professional's duty to protect a young person from serious harm will outweigh their duty to maintain confidentiality, although each case should be considered in its own right.

References

Action for Children and New Economics Foundation (2009). *Backing the Future: why investing in children is good for us all*. London: Action for Children/NEF.

Adams, S., Kuebli, J., Boyle, P. and Fivush, R. (1995). Gender differences in parent–child conversations about past emotions: a longitudinal investigation. *Sex Roles*, 33(5–6), 309–23.

Ainscough, C. and Toon, K. (1998). *Breaking Free: help for survivors of child sexual abuse*. London: Sheldon Press.

Allard, R., Marshall, M. and Plante, M. (1992). Intensive follow up does not decrease the risk of repeat suicide attempts. *Suicide Life Threatening Behaviours*, (22), 302–14.

Altschul, A. (1997). A personal view of psychiatric nursing. In Tilley, S. (ed) *The Mental Health Nurse: views of practice and education*. Oxford: Blackwell Science.

American Psychiatric Association (1994). *Diagnostic and Statistical Manual of Mental Disorders* (4th edition). Washington, DC: APA.

Anderson, M., Armstrong, M., Armstrong, S., Nadkarni, A. and Pluck, G. (2009). *Self Harm and Repeat Self Harm in Young People: a comparative study of social and psychological factors*. Not yet published.

Anderson, M., Woodward, L. and Armstrong, M. (2004). Self harm in young people: a perspective for mental health nursing care. *International Nursing Review*, 51, 222–8.

Angold, A. (1994). Clinical interviewing with children and adolescents. In Rutter, M., Taylor, E. and Hersov, L. (eds) *Child and Adolescent Psychiatry: modern approaches* (3rd edition). London: Blackwell.

Antretter, E., Dunkel, D., Haring, C., Corcoran, P., De Leo, D., Fekete, S., Hawton, K., Kerkhof, A. J. F. M., Lonnqvist, J., Salander Renberg, E., Schmidtke, A., Van Heeringen, K. and Wasserman, D. (2008). The factorial structure of the Suicidal Intent Scale: a comparative study in clinical samples from 11 European regions. *International Journal of Methods in Psychiatric Research*, (7), 63–79.

Armstrong, M. (1995). The Management of Self–harm in Children and Adolescents. Unpublished thesis: University of Lancaster.

Armstrong, M. (2006). Self harm, young people and nursing. In McDougall, T. (ed) *Child and Adolescent Mental Health Nursing*. London: Blackwell Publishing.

Arnold, L. (1995). *Women and Self Injury: a survey of 76 women. A report on women's experience of self injury and their views on service provision*. Bristol: Bristol Crisis Service for Women.

Asarow, J., Carlson, G. and Guthrie, D. (1987). Coping strategies, self perceptions, hopelessness and perceived family environments in depressed and suicidal children. *Journal of Consulting and Clinical Psychiatry*, (55), 361–6.

Asen, E. (2002). Outcome research in family therapy. *Advances in Psychiatric Treatment*, (8), 230–8.

Austin, L. and Kortum, J. (1996). Self injury: the secret language of pain for teenagers. *Education*, 22 March 2004.

Avan, G. and Bakshi, N. (2004). *Young Black and Ethnic Minority Women and Self Esteem: a report to the Glasgow Anti–Racist Alliance*. Glasgow: Glasgow Anti Racist Alliance.

Babiker, G. and Arnold, L. (1997). *The Language of Injury: comprehending self mutilation*. Leicester: BPS Books.

Baker, D. and Fortune, S. (2008). Understanding self–harm and suicide websites. *Crisis: Journal of Crisis Intervention and Suicide Prevention*, 29(3), 118–22.

Barish, K. (2004). What is therapeutic in child therapy? Therapeutic engagement. *Psychoanalytic Psychology*, 21, 385–401.

Barker, P. (2004). *Assessment in Psychiatric and Mental Health Nursing: in search of the whole person*. Cheltenham: Nelson Thornes.

Barley, W., Buie, S., Peterson, E., Hollingsworth, A., Griva, M., Hickerson, S., Lawson, J. and Bailey, B. (1993). Development of an in–patient cognitive behavioural treatment programme for borderline personality disorder. *Journal of Personality Disorders*, 7(3), 232–40.

Barnardo's and Mind (2007). *About Self Harm: a guide for young people: when you self harm and how to seek help*. London: Barnardo's.

Basement Project (1997). *What's the Harm? A book for young people who self harm or self injure*. Manchester: Lois Arnold and Anne Magill.

Bates, T. (2005). 'Suicide Prevention: everyone's problem'. Summary of the Forum for Integration and Partnership of Stakeholders in Suicide Prevention: Dublin.

Beautrais, A. (2001). Child and young adolescent suicide in New Zealand. *Australian and New Zealand Journal of Psychiatry*, 35(5), 647–53.

Beautrais, A., Joyce, P. and Mulder, R. (1998). Psychiatric illness in a New Zealand sample of young people making serious suicide attempts. *New Zealand Medical Journal*, 27, 44–8.

Beck, A., Steer, A. and Beck, K. (1993). Hopelessness, depression, suicidal ideation and clinical diagnosis of depression. *Suicide and Life Threatening Behavior*, 23(2), 139–45.

Bennewith, O., Hawton, K., Simkin, S., Sutton, L., Kapur, N., Turnbull, P. and Gunnell, D. (2005). The usefulness of coroners' data on suicides for providing information relevant to prevention. *Suicide and Life Threatening Behavior*, (35), 607–14.

Bennewith, O., Stocks, N. and Gunnell, D. (2002). General practice based intervention to prevent repeat episodes of deliberate self harm: cluster randomised controlled trial. *British Medical Journal*, (324), 1254–7.

Bergen, H., Hawton, K., Murphy, E., Cooper, J., Kapur, N., Stalker, C. and Waters, K. (2009). Trends in prescribing and self–poisoning in relation to UK regulatory authority warnings against use of SSRI antidepressants in under–18–year–olds. *British Journal of Clinical Pharmacology*, (68), 618–29.

Berman, A. and Carroll, T. (1984). Adolescent suicide: a critical review. *Death Studies*, (8), 53–63.

Bernstein, D., Cohen, P. and Velez, C. (1993). Prevalence and stability of the *DSM–III–R* personality disorders in a community based survey of adolescents. *American Journal of Psychiatry*, (150), 1237–43.

Best, R. (2005). Self Harm: a challenge for pastoral care. *Pastoral Care in Education*, 23(3), 3–11.

Bhugra, D., Thompson, N., Singh, J. and Fellow–Smith, E. (2004). Deliberate self harm in adolescents in West London: socio–cultural factors. *European Journal of Psychiatry*, 18(2), 91–8.

Biddle, L., Donovan, J., Hawton, K., Kapur, N. and Gunnell, D. (2008). Suicide and the internet. *British Medical Journal*, (336), 800–2.

Bille–Brahe, U., Kerkhof, A., De Leo, D. and Schmidtke, A. (2004). Definitions and terminology used in the WHO/EURO Multicentre study in Suicidal Behaviour in Europe: Results from the WHO/EURO Multicentre Study on Suicidal Behaviour, 1, 11–14, Schmidtke, A., Bille–Brahe, U., De Leo, D. and Kerkhof, A. (eds) Australian Institute for Suicide Research and Prevention.

Black, D. (1992). Mental health services for children. *British Medical Journal*, (305), 971–2.

Blood, R., Pirkis, J. and Holland, K. (2007). Media reporting of suicide methods. *Crisis*, 28(1), 64–9.

Blumenthal, S. and Kupfer, D. (1990). *Suicide over the Life Cycle*. Washington, DC: American Psychiatric Press.

Bohus, M., Haaf, B., Stiglmayr, C., Pohl, U., Bohme, R. and Linehan, M. (2001). Evaluation of in–patient dialectical behavioural therapy for borderline personality disorder: a prospective study. *Behavior Research and Therapy*, (38), 875–87.

Bond, F. and Bruch, M. (1998). *Beyond Diagnosis: case formulation approaches in CBT*. New York: Wiley.

Bracken, K., Berman, M., McCloskey, M. and Bullock, J. (2008). Deliberate self harm and state dissociation: an experimental investigation. *Journal of Aggression, Maltreatment and Trauma*, 17(4), 520–32.

Bradley, K. (2009). *The Bradley Report: review of people with mental health problems or learning disabilities in the criminal justice system*. London: HMSO.

Brent, D. (1997). Practitioner Review: the aftercare of adolescents with deliberate self–harm. *Journal of Child Psychology and Psychiatry*, 38(3), 277–86.

Brent, D., Bridge, J. and Johnson, B. (1996). Suicidal behaviour runs in families: a controlled family study of adolescent suicide victims. *Archives of General Psychiatry*, 53(12), 1145–52.

Brent, D., Holder, D., Kolko, D., Birmaher, B., Braugher, M. and Roth C. (1997). A clinical psychotherapy trial for adolescent depression comparing cognitive, family and supportive treatments. *Archives of General Psychiatry*, (54), 877–85.

Brent, D., Kerr, M., Goldstein, C., Bozigar, J., Wartella, M. and Allan, M. (1989). An outbreak of suicide and suicidal behaviour in high school. *Journal of the American Academy of Child and Adolescent Psychiatry*, (28), 918–24.

Brent, D., Perper, J., Mortiz, G., Baugher, M., Schweers, J. and Roth, C. (1994). Suicide in affectively ill adolescents: a case control study. *Journal of Affective Disorders*, 31(3), 193–202.

British Medical Association (2003). *Adolescent Health*. London: BMA.

Brodie, I., Berridge, D. and Beckett, W. (1997). The health of children looked after by local authorities. *British Journal of Nursing*, 6(7), 386–90.

Brown, J., Cohen, P., Johnson, J. and Smaile, E. (1999). Childhood abuse and neglect: specificity of effects on adolescent and young adult depression and suicidality. *American Academy of Child and Adolescent Psychiatry*, 38(12), 1490–6.

Brown, R. (2002). Self harm and suicide risk for same sex attracted young people: a family perspective. *Australian e–journal for the Advancement of Mental Health*, 1(1).

Burke, M., Duffy, D., Trainor, G. and Shinner, M. (2008) *Self injury toolkit*, Manchester: Greater Manchester West Mental Health Foundation Trust.

Byrne, S., Morgan, S., Fitzpatrick, C., Boylan, C., Crowley, S., Gahan, H., Howley, J., Staunton, D. and Guerin, S. (2008). Deliberate self–harm in children and adolescents: a qualitative study exploring the needs of parents and carers. *Clinical Psychology and Psychiatry*, October, 13(4), 493–504.

Bywaters, P. and Rolfe, A. (2002). *Look Beyond the Scars: understanding and responding to self injury and self harm*. London: NCH.

Carter, G., Clover, K. and Whyte, I. (2005). Postcards from the Edge project: randomised controlled trial of an intervention using postcards to reduce repetition of hospital treated deliberate self poisoning. *British Medical Journal*, (331), 805.

Cathcart, B. (2007). Deepcut: the media messed up. *British Journalism Review*, 18(1), 7–12.

Centers for Disease Control (1990). Attempted suicide among high school students – United States 1990. *Morbidity and Mortality Weekly Report (MMWR)* 1991, 40, 633–5.

Centers for Disease Control (1992). *Youth Suicide Prevention Programs: a resource guide.* Atlanta: US Department of Health and Human Services.

Cheng, A. T. A., Hawton, K., Chen, T. H. H., Yen, A. M. F., Chang, J.–C., Chong, M.–Y., Liu, C.–Y., Lee, Y., Teng, P.–R., Chen, L.–C. (2007a). The influence of media reporting of a celebrity suicide on suicidal behaviour in patients with a history of depressive disorder. *Journal of Affective Disorders*, (103), 69–75.

Cheng, A. T. A., Hawton, K., Chen, T. H. H., Yen, A. M. F., Chen, C.–Y., Chen, L.–C., Teng, P.–R. (2007b). The influence of media coverage of a celebrity suicide on subsequent suicide attempts. *Journal of Clinical Psychiatry*, (68), 862–6.

Children's Society (2009). *A Good Childhood: searching for values in a competitive age.* London: Children's Society.

Chitsabesan, P., Harrington, R., Harrington, V. and Tomenson, B. (2003). Predicting repeat self–harm in children. How accurate can we expect to be? *European Child and Adolescent Psychiatry*, 12, 23–9.

Chowdhury, N., Hicks, R. and Kreitman, N. (1973). Evaluation of an after care service for parasuicide (attempted suicide) patients. *Social Psychiatry and Psychiatric Epidemiology*, (8), 67–81.

Christofferson, M., Poulsen, H. and Nielson, A. (2003). Attempted suicide among young people: risk factors in a prospective register based study of Danish children born in 1966. *Acta Psychiatrica Scandinavica*, 108(5), 350–8.

Clark, T., Sherr, L. and Watts, C. (2000). *Young People and Self Harm: pathways in care.* Public Health Research Report 140. Barking and Havering Health Authority. Public Health Directorate.

Clarke, J. (2003). *Women's Experiences of Attending a Self Harm Self Help Group.* Unpublished work.

Coleman, J., Hendry, L. and Kloep, M. (2007). *Adolescence and Health.* London: Wiley.

Cotgrove, A. (2005). Depression and self harm. In Gowers, S. (ed) *Seminars in Child and Adolescent Psychiatry.* (2nd edition). London: Gaskell.

Cotgrove, A. (2007). Should young people be given antidepressants? – Yes. *British Medical Journal*, (335), 750.

Cotgrove, A., McLaughlin, R., O'Herlihy, A. and Lelliot, P. (2007). The ability of adolescent psychiatric units to accept emergency admissions: changes in England and Wales between 2000 and 2005. *Psychiatric Bulletin*, (31), 457–9.

Cotgrove, A., Zirinsky, L., Black, D. and Weston, D. (1995). Secondary prevention of attempted suicide in adolescence. *Journal of Adolescence*, (18), 569–77.

Cousins, W., McGowan, I. and Milner, S. (2008). Self harm and attempted suicide in young people looked after in state care. *Journal of Children's and Young People's Nursing*, 2(2), 51–4.

Cowdery, G., Iwata, B. and Pace, G. (1990). Effects and side effects of DRO as treatment for self–injurious behavior. *Journal of Applied Behavioral Analysis*, (23), 497–506.

Crawford, M. (1998). Deliberate self harm assessment by accident and emergency staff: an interventional study. *Journal of Accident and Emergency Medicine*, 15(1), 18–20.

Cullen, J. (2006). *Meanings, Messages and Myths: the coverage and treatment of suicide in the Irish print media.* Dublin: National Office for Suicide Prevention.

Daniel, B. and Wassell, S. (2002). *Assessing and Promoting Resilience in Vulnerable Children.* London: Jessica Kingsley Publishers.

de Wilde, E., Kienhorst, I. and Diekstra, R. (2001). Suicidal behaviour in adolescents. In Goodyer, I. (ed) *The Depressed Child and Adolescent* (2nd edition). London: Cambridge University Press.

Dennehy, J., Appelby, L. and Thomas, C. (1996). Case control study of suicide by discharged psychiatric patients. *British Medical Journal*, 312(7046), 1580.

Department for Children, Schools and Families (2008). T*he Children Act 1989: guidance and regulations. Volume 1: court orders.* London: TSO.

Department For Education and Skills (2002). *Bullying: don't suffer in silence.* London: HMSO.

Department for Education and Skills (2003). *Every Child Matters.* London: HMSO.

Department for Education and Skills (2005a). *Excellence and Enjoyment: social and emotional aspects of learning.* London: TSO.

Department for Education and Skills (2005b). *National Healthy Schools Status: a guide for schools.* London: TSO.

Department for Education and Skills (2006a). *Working Together to Safeguard Children: a guide to interagency working to safeguard and promote the welfare of children.* London: HMSO.

Department for Education and Skills (2006b). *Information Sharing: practitioners guide.* London: HMSO.

Department of Health (1999). *Saving Lives: our healthier nation.* London: HMSO.

Department of Health (2002a). *National Suicide Prevention Strategy for England.* London: HMSO.

Department of Health (2002b). *Women's Mental Health: Into the Mainstream: strategic development of mental health care for women.* London: HMSO.

Department of Health (2003). *Confidentiality: NHS Code of Practice.* London: HMSO.

Department of Health (2004). *National Service Framework for Children, Young People and Maternity Services.* London: HMSO.

Department of Health (2006). *Standards for Better Health.* London: HMSO.

Department of Health (2007a). *Best Practice in Managing Risk: principles and guidance for best practice in the assessment and management of risk to self and others in mental health services.* London: HMSO.

Department of Health (2007b). *Promoting Mental Health for Children Held in Secure Settings: a framework for commissioning service*s. London: HMSO.

Department of Health (2008). *Refocusing the Care Programme Approach.* London: HMSO.

Department of Health (2009). *Healthy Lives, Brighter Futures: the strategy for children and young people's health.* London: HMSO.

Department of Health and Children (1999). *Report of the National Task Force on Suicide.* Dublin: Stationary Office.

Department of Health, Social Services and Public Safety (2001). *Review of Nursing, Midwifery and Health Visiting Workforce: report of KPMG consulting and DHSSPS nursing and midwifery workforce planning initiative steering group.* Belfast: DHSSPS.

Department of Health, Social Services and Public Safety (2003). *Promoting Mental Health: strategy and action plan 2003–8.* Belfast: DHSSPS.

Diekstra, R. (1995). Depression and suicidal behaviours in adolescence: sociocultural and time trends. In Rutter, M. (ed) *Psychosocial Disturbances in Young People.* Cambridge: Cambridge University Press.

Diekstra, R. and Hawton, K. (1987). *Suicide in Adolescence.* Dordrecht/Canberra: Kluwer Academic Publishers.

Dimeff, L., Koerner, K. and Linehan, M. (2002). *Summary of Research on Dialectical Behaviour Therapy.* Seattle: The Behavioral Technology Transfer Group.

Dorer, C. (1998). An evaluation of protocols for child and adolescent deliberate self harm. *Child Psychology and Psychiatry Review*, 3(4), 156–60.

Dow, P. (2004). *I Feel Like I'm Invisible: children talking to ChildLine about self harm*. London: Mental Health Foundation and Camelot Foundation.

Eddleston, M., Sheriff, M. and Hawton, K. (1998). Deliberate self harm in Sri Lanka: an overlooked tragedy in the developing world. *British Medical Journal*, (317), 133–5.

Edwards, L. (2003). *Promoting Young People's Wellbeing: a review of research on emotional health*. SCRE Centre: University of Glasgow.

Edwards, V. (2007). Therapeutic issues in working individually with vulnerable children and young people. In Vostanis, P. (ed) *Mental Health Interventions and Services for Vulnerable Children and Young People*. London: Jessica Kingsley Publishers.

Egmond, M. and van Diekstra, R. (1989). The predictability of suicidal behaviour: the results of a meta–analysis of published studies. In Diekstra, R., Platt, S., Schmidt, K. and Sonneck, G. (eds) *Suicide Prevention: the role of attitude and imitation*. The Netherlands: Leides.

Emerson, L. (1913). The case of Miss A: a preliminary report of a psychoanalysis study and the treatment of a case of self mutilation. *Psychoanalytic Review*, (1), 41–54.

Erikson, E. (1968). *Identity, Youth and Crisis*. New York: Norton.

Evans, J., Platts, H. and Liebenau, A. (1996). Impulsiveness and deliberate self harm: a comparison of 'first timers' and 'repeaters'. *Acta Scandinavica Psychiactrica*, 93(5), 378–80.

Evans, K., Tyrer, P. and Catalan, J. (1999). Manual assisted cognitive behaviour therapy (MACT): a randomised controlled trial of a brief intervention with bibliotherapy in the treatment of recurrent deliberate self harm. *Psychological Medicine*, (29), 19–25.

Fagin, L. (2006). Repeated self injury: perspectives from general psychiatry. *Advances in Psychiatric Treatment*, 12, 193–201.

Faith, K. (2002). Addressing issues of autonomy and beneficence in the treatment of eating disorders. Available at www.nedic.ca.

Farber, S. (2008). Dissociation, traumatic attachments, and self harm: eating disorders and self mutilation. *Clinical Social Work Journal*, 36(1), 63–72.

Farley, A., Hendry, C. and Napier, P. (2005). Paracetamol and poisoning: physiological aspects and management strategies. *Nursing Standard*, 19(38), 58–64.

Favaro, A. and Santonastaso, P. (2000). Self injurious behaviour in anorexia nervosa. *Journal of Nervous and Mental Disease*, 188(8), 537–42.

Favazza, A. (1996). *Bodies Under Siege: self mutilation and body modification in culture and psychiatry*. New York: Johns Hopkins University Press.

Favazza, A. (1998). The coming of age of self mutilation. *Journal of Nervous and Mental Disease*, 186(5), 259–68.

Favazza, A., DeRosear, L. and Conterio, K. (1989). Self mutilation and eating disorders. *Suicide and Life Threatening Behaviour*, 19(4), 352–61.

Favazza, A. and Rosenthal, R. (1993). Diagnostic issues in self mutilation. *Hospital and Community Psychiatry*, 44, 134–40.

Fivush, R., Brotma, M., Buckner, J. and Goodman, S. (2004). Parent–child emotion narratives. *Sex Roles*, 42(3–4), 233–53.

Fonagy, P. (2003). *A review of the outcomes of all treatments of psychiatric disorder in childhood: (MCH 17–33)*. London: HMSO.

Fonagy, P., Target, M., Cottrell, D., Phillips, J. and Kurtz, Z. (2002). *What Works for Whom? a critical review of treatments for children and adolescents*. London: Guilford Press.

Fortune, S., Sinclair, J. and Hawton, K. (2005). *Adolescents' views on prevention of self harm, barriers to help seeking for self harm and how quality of life might be improved: a qualitative and quantitative study*. University of Oxford: Centre for Suicide Research.

Fox, C. and Hawton, K. (2004). *Deliberate Self Harm in Adolescence*. London: Jessica Kingsley Publishers.

Gale, F. (2007). Tackling the stigma of mental health in vulnerable children and young people. In Vostanis, P. (ed) *Mental Health Interventions and Services for Vulnerable Children and Young People*. London: Jessica Kingsley Publishers.

Garcia, I., Vasiliou, C. and Penketh, K. (2007). *Listen up!: person centred approaches to help young people experiencing mental health and emotional problems*. London: Mental Health Foundation.

Garthwaite, T. (2009). Trial by Media. *YoungMinds*, (100), 16–17.

Gibbons, J., Butler, J., Urwin, P. and Gibbons, J. (1978). Evaluation of a social work service for self poisoning patients. *British Journal of Psychiatry*, (133), 111–18.

Gilbert, P., Gilbert, J. and Sanghera, J. (2004). A focus group exploration of the impact of izzat, shame, subordination and entrapment on mental health and service use in South Asian women living in Derby. *Mental Health, Religion and Culture*, 7(2), 109–30.

Gispert, M., Davis, M., Marsh, L. and Wheeler, K. (1987). Predictive factors in repeated suicide attempts by adolescents. *Hospital Community Psychiatry*, (38), 390–3.

Gladstone, G., Parker, G., Mitchell, P., Malhi, G., Wilhelm, K. and Austin, M. (2004). Implications of childhood trauma for depressed women: an analysis of pathways from childhood sexual abuse to deliberate self harm and revictimization. *American Journal of Psychiatry*, (161), 1417–25.

Glasgow Violence Against Women Partnership. (2008). *Self Harm and Suicide Among Black and Minority Ethnic Women*. Glasgow: GVAWP.

Goffman, E. (1963). *Stigma: notes on the management of spoiled identity*. Englewood Cliffs, NJ: Prentice Hall.

Goldacre, M. and Hawton, K. (1988). Repetition of self poisoning and subsequent death in adolescents who take overdoses. *British Journal of Psychiatry*, (146), 395–8.

Goodman, R. (1997). The strengths and difficulties questionnaire: a research note. *Journal of Child Psychology and Psychiatry*, 38, 581–6.

Goodyer, I., Dubicka, B., Wilkinson, P., Kelvin, R., Roberts, C., Byford, S., Breen, S., Ford, C., Barrett, B., Leech, A., Rothwell, J., White, L. and Harrington, R. (2007). Selective serotonin reuptake inhibitors (SSRIs) and routine specialist care with and without cognitive behaviour therapy in adolescents with major depression: randomised controlled trial. *British Medical Journal*, 335, 142.

Gosney, H. and Hawton, K. (2007). Inquest verdicts: youth suicides lost. *Psychiatric Bulletin*, 31, 203–5.

Gould, M. (2001). *Suicide and the Media*. Annals. New York: New York Academy of Sciences.

Gould, M., Greenberg, T. and Velting, D. (2003). Youth suicide risk and preventive interventions: a review of the past 10 years. *Journal of the American Academy of Child and Adolescent Psychiatry*, (42), 386–405.

Gould, M., Wallenstein, S. and Kleinman, M. (1990). Time–space clustering of teenage suicide. *American Journal of Epidemiology*, (131), 71–8.

Gowers, S., Harrington, R. and Whitton, A. (1998). *Health of the Nation Outcome Scales for Children and Adolescents (HoNOSCA)*. London: Royal College of Psychiatrists Research Unit.

Gowers, S., Thomas, S. and Deeley, S. (2004). Can primary schools contribute effectively to Tier 1 child mental health services? *Clinical Child Psychology and Psychiatry*, (9), 419–25.

Granboulan, V., Rabain, D. and Basquin, M. (1995). The outcome of adolescent suicide attempts. *Acta Psychiatrica Scandinavica*, (91), 265–70.

Green, A. (1978). Self destructive behavior in battered children. *American Journal of Psychiatry*, (135), 579–82.

Green, H., McGinnity, A., Meltzer, H., Ford, T. and Goodman, R. (2005). *Mental health of children and young people in Great Britain*. London: ONS.

Green, J., Wood, A., Kerfoot, M., Trainor, G., Roberts, C., Rothwell, J., Woodham, A., Ayodeji, E., Barret, B. and Byford, S. (2010). Group Therapeutic Treatment for Adolescents with repeated self harm ASSIST – a randomised controlled trial with economic evaluation. *British Medical Journal* (forthcoming, summer 2010).

Gross, E. (2004). Adolescent internet use: what we expect, what teens report. *Journal of Applied Developmental Psychology*, (25), 633–49.

Gunnell, D. (1994). *The Potential for Preventing Suicide: a review of the literature on the effectiveness of interventions aimed at preventing suicide.* Bristol HCEU. University of Bristol.

Gunnell, D. and Frankel, S. (1994). Prevention of suicide: aspirations and evidence. *British Medical Journal*, (308), 1227–33.

Gunnell, D., Hawton, K., Ho, D., Evans, J., O'Connor, S., Potokar, J., Donovan, J. and Kapur, N. (2008). Hospital admissions for self–harm following psychiatric hospital discharge: cohort study. *British Medical Journal*, (337), 1331–4.

Gunnell, D., Platt, S. and Hawton, K. (2009). The economic crisis and suicide: consequences may be serious and warrant early attention. *British Medical Journal*, (338), 1456–7.

Harbour, A. (2008). *Children with Mental Disorder and the Law: a guide to law and practice.* London: Jessica Kingsley Publishers.

Harden, A., Rees, A. and Shepherd, J. (2003). *Young People and Mental Health: a systematic review of research on barriers and facilitators.* London: EPPI Centre.

Hargus, E., Hawton, K. and Rodham, K. (2009). Distinguishing between subgroups of adolescents who self harm. *Suicide and Life Threatening Behavior*, (39), 518–37.

Harrington, R. (2001). Depression, suicide and deliberate self–harm in adolescence. *British Medical Bulletin*, 57, 47–60.

Harrington, R., Whittaker, J., Shoebridge, P. and Campbell, F. (1998a). Systematic review of efficacy of cognitive behaviour therapies in child and adolescent depressive disorder. *British Medical Journal*, 316, 1559–63.

Harrington, R., Kerfoot, M., Dyer, E., McNiven, F., Gill, J., Harrington, V., Woodham, A. and Byford, S. (1998b). Randomised trial of a home based family intervention for children who have deliberately poisoned themselves. *Journal of the American Academy of Child Adolescent Psychiatry*, (37), 512–18.

Hawton, K. (1986). *Suicide and Attempted Suicide among Children and Adolescents.* Beverley Hills, CA: Sage.

Hawton, K. (1992). Trends in deliberate self poisoning and self injury in Oxford. *British Medical Journal*, (304), 1409–11.

Hawton, K. (2002). United Kingdom legislation on pack sizes of analgesics: background, rationale and effects on suicide and deliberate self harm. *Suicide and Life Threatening Behavior*, 32(3), 223–9.

Hawton, K. (2005). *Prevention and Treatment of Suicidal Behaviour: from science to practice.* London: Oxford University Press.

Hawton, K., Arensman, E., Townsend, E., Bremner, S., Feldman, E., Goldney, R., Gunnell, D., Hazell, P., van Heeringen, K., House, A., Owens, D., Sakinofsky, I. and Träskman–Bendz, L. (1998b). Deliberate self harm: systematic review of efficacy of psychosocial and pharmacological treatments in preventing repetition. *British Medical Journal*, 317, 441–7.

Hawton, K., Arensman, E., Wasserman, D., Hulten, A. and Bille–Brane, U. (1998a). Relation between suicide and attempted suicide rates among young people in Europe. *Journal of Epidemiology and Community Health*, (52), 191–4.

Hawton, K., Bankcroft, J., Catalan, J., Kingston, B., Stedeford, A. and Welch, N. (1981). Domiciliary and outpatient treatment of self poisoning patients by medical and non medical staff. *Psychological Medicine* (11), 169–77.

Hawton, K. and Catalan, J. (1987). *Attempted Suicide: a practical guide to its nature and management.* (2nd edition). Oxford: Oxford Medical Publications.

Hawton, K. and Fagg, J. (1992). Deliberate self–poisoning and injury in adolescents: a study of characteristics and trends in Oxford 1976–89. *British Journal of Psychiatry*, 161, 816–23.

Hawton, K., Fagg, J., Simkin, S., Harris, L., Bale, E. and Bond, A. (1996). Deliberate self poisoning and self injury in children and adolescents under 16 years of age in Oxford 1976–93. *British Journal of Psychiatry*, (169), 202–8.

Hawton, K., Hall, S., Simkin, S., Bale, S., Bond, A., Codd, S. and Stewart, A. (2003). Deliberate self harm in adolescents: a study of characteristics and trends in Oxford, 1990–2000. *Journal of Child Psychology and Psychiatry*, 44(8), 1191–8.

Hawton, K. and Harriss, L. (2008). Deliberate self harm by under 15 year olds: characteristics, trends and outcome. *Journal of Child Psychology and Psychiatry*, 49(4), 441–8.

Hawton, K., Harriss, L., Appleby, L., Juszczak, E., Simkin, S., McDonnell, R., Amos, T., Kiernan, K. and Parrott, H. (2000). Death of the Princess of Wales and subsequent suicide and self–harm. *British Journal of Psychiatry*, (177), 463–6.

Hawton, K. and James, A. (2005). ABC of adolescence: suicide and deliberate self harm in young people. *British Medical Journal*, 330(16), 891–4.

Hawton, K. and Kirk, J. (1989). Problem solving. In Hawton, P., Salkovskis, P. and Kirk, J. (eds) *Cognitive Behaviour Therapy for Psychiatric Problems: a practical guide.* Oxford: Oxford Medical Publications.

Hawton, K., McKeown, S., Day, A., Martin, P., O'Connor, M. and Yule, J. (1987). Evaluation of outpatient counselling compared with general practitioner care following overdoses. *Psychological Medicine*, (17), 751–61.

Hawton, K., Osborn, M., O'Grady, J. and Cole, D. (1982). Adolescents who take overdoses: their characteristics, problems and contacts with helping agencies. *British Journal of Psychiatry*, (140), 118–23.

Hawton, K., Ratnayeke, L., Simkin, S., Harriss, L. and Scott, V. (2009). Evaluation of acceptability and use of lockable storage devices for pesticides in Sri Lanka that might assist in prevention of self–poisoning. *BMC Public Health*, (9), 69.

Hawton, K. and Rodham, K. (2006). *By Their Own Young Hand: deliberate self harm and suicidal ideas in adolescents.* London: Jessica Kingsley Publishers.

Hawton, K., Rodham, K., Evans, E. and Weatherall, R. (2002). Deliberate self harm in adolescents: self report survey in schools in England. *British Medical Journal*, (325), 1207–11.

Hawton, K. and Simkin, S. (2008). *Help is at Hand.* London. Department of Health Publications.

Hawton, K., Simkin, S. and Deeks, J. (1999). Effects of a drug overdose in a television drama on presentations to hospital for self poisoning: time series and questionnaire study. *British Medical Journal*, (318), 972–7.

Hawton, K., Sutton, L., Haw, C., Sinclair, J. and Deeks, J. (2005). Schizophrenia and suicide: systematic review of risk factors. *British Journal of Psychiatry*, 187, 9–20.

Hawton, K., Townsend, E., Deeks, J., Appleby, L., Gunnell, D., Bennewith, O. and Cooper, J. (2001). Effects of legislation restricting pack sizes of paracetamol and salicylates on self poisoning in the United Kingdom: before and after study *British Medical Journal*, (322), 1203–7.

Hepp, U., Wittmann, L. and Schnyder, U. (2004). Psychological and psychosocial interventions after attempted suicide: an overview of treatment studies. *Crisis*, (25), 108–17.

Hill, P. and Taylor, E. (2001). An auditable protocol for treating attention deficit hyperactivity disorder. *Archives of Disease in Childhood*, (84), 404–9.

Hirsch, S., Walsh, C., and Draper, R. (1982). Parasuicide: a review of treatment interventions. *Journal of Affective Disorders*, (4), 299–311.

HM Government (2008). *Staying Safe: action plan.* London: HMSO.

HM Inspectorate of Prisons (2007). *The Mental Health of Prisoners: a thematic review of the care and support of prisoners with mental health needs.* London: HMPI.

HM Treasury (2008). *Safeguarding Children: the 3rd Joint Chief Inspectors Report on Arrangements to Safeguard Children.* London: HMSO.

Hodkinson, P. (2002). *Goth: identity, style and subculture.* Oxford: Berg.

Horowitz, L., Wang, P., Koocher, G. and Burr, B. (2001). Detecting Suicide Risk in a Pediatric Emergency Department: development of a brief screening tool. *Pediatrics*, 107(5), 1133–8.

Huband, N., McMurran, M. and Evans, C. (2007). Social problem solving plus psycho education for adults with personality disorder: pragmatic randomised controlled trial. *British Journal of Psychiatry*, 190, 307–13.

Huey, S., Henggeler, S., Rowland, M., Halliday–Boykins, C., Cunningham, P. and Pickrel, S. (2004). Multi systemic therapy effects on attempted suicide by youths presenting psychiatric emergencies. *Journal of the American Academy of Child and Adolescent Psychiatry*, 43(2), 183–90.

Hurry, J. and Storey, P. (1998). *Deliberate self harm among young people.* London: Institute of Education.

Institute of Alcohol Studies. (2006). *Fact sheet: adolescents and alcohol.* Cambridge: IAS.

Iverson, C. (2002). Solution focused brief therapy. *Advances in Psychiatric Treatment*, (8), 149–57.

Jamieson, K. and Hawton, K. (2005). The burden of suicide and clinical suggestions for prevention. In Hawton, K. (ed) *Prevention and Treatment of Suicidal Behaviour: from science to practice.* Oxford: Oxford University Press.

Jones, D. (2003). *Communicating with Vulnerable Children: a guide for practitioners.* London: Gaskell.

Jones, M. and Jones, D. (1995). Preferred pathways of behavioural contagion. *Journal of Psychiatric Research*, (29), 193–209.

Juhnke, G. (1994). The adapted SAD PERSONS: a suicide assessment scale designed for use with children. *Elementary School Guidance and Counseling*, 30(4), 252–8.

Juhnke, G. (1996). SAD PERSONS Scale review. *Measurement in Counseling and Development*, 27(1), 325–7.

Kahan, J. and Pattison, E. (1984). Proposal for a distinctive diagnosis: the deliberate self harm syndrome. *Suicide and Life Threatening Behavior*, (14), 17–35.

Kaledienne, R., Starkuvienne, S. and Petrauskiene, J. (2006). Seasonal patterns of suicides over the period of socio–economic transition in Lithuania. *BMC Public Health*, 22(6), 40.

Kapur, N., Cooper, J. and Hiroeh, U. (2004a). Emergency department management and outcome for self–poisoning: a cohort study. *General Hospital Psychiatry*, (26), 36–41.

Kapur, N., Cooper, J., Rodway, C., Kelly, J. and Mackway–Jones, K. (2004b). Predicting the risk of repetition after self harm. *British Medical Journal*, 330(7488), 394–5.

Kapur, N., House, A. and Dodgson, K. (2002). Effect of general hospital management on repeat episodes of deliberate self harm poisoning: cohort study. *British Medical Journal*, (325), 866–7.

Kapur, N., Murphy, E., Cooper, J., Bergen, H., Hawton, K., Simkin, S., Casey, D., Horrocks, J., Lilley, R., Noble, R. and Owens, D. (2008). Psychosocial assessment following self–harm: results from the Multi Centre Monitoring of Self Harm Project. *Journal of Affective Disorders*, (106), 285–93.

Kendall–Tackett, K., Williams, L. and Finkelhor, D. (1993). Impact of sexual abuse of children: a review and synthesis of recent empirical studies. *Psychological Bulletin*, 113(1), 164–80.

Kerfoot, M. (1988). Deliberate self poisoning in childhood and early adolescence. *Journal of Child Psychology and Psychiatry*, 29, 335–43.

Kerfoot, M. (2000). Youth suicide and deliberate self harm. In Aggleton, P., Hurry, J. and Warwick, I. (eds) *Young People and Mental Health.* Chichester. John Wiley and Sons.

Kerfoot, M., Dyer, E., Harrington, V., Woodham, A. and Harrington, R. (1996). Correlates and short–term course of self–poisoning in adolescents. *British Journal of Psychiatry*, 168, 38–42.

Kerfoot, M., Dyer, E., Harrington, V., Woodham, A. and Harrington, R. (1996). Correlates and short term course of self poisoning in adolescents. *British Journal of Psychiatry*, (68), 38–42.

Kerfoot, M., Harrington, R. and Dyer, E. (1995). Brief home based intervention with young suicide attempters and their families. *Journal of Adolescence*, 18(5), 557–68.

Kessel, N. and Grossman, G. (1961). Suicide in alcoholics: alcohol and road accidents. *British Medical Journal*, (2), 1671–2.

Kienhorst, C., Wolters, W., Diekstra, R. and Otte, E. (1987). A study of the frequency of suicidal behaviour in children aged 5 to 14. *Journal of Child Psychology and Psychiatry*, (28), 153–65.

Kingsbury, S. (1993). Clinical components of suicidal intent in adolescent overdose. *Journal of American Academy of Child and Adolescent Psychiatry*, 32(3), 518–20.

Kingsbury, S. (1996). PATHOS: a screening instrument for adolescent overdose: a research note. *Journal of Psychology and Psychiatry*, (37), 609–11.

Kingsbury, S., Hawton, K., Steinhardt, D. and James, A. (1999). Do adolescents who take overdoses have specific psychological characteristics? A comparative study with psychiatric and community controls. *Journal of American Academy of Child and Adolescent Psychiatry*, 38, 1125–31.

Kingston, B., Regoli, B. and Hewitt, J. (2004). The theory of differential oppression: a developmental–ecological explanation of adolescent problem behaviour. *Critical Criminology*, 11(3), 237–60.

Kloep, M. and Hendry, L. (1999). Challenges, risks and coping in adolescence. In Messer, D. and Millar, S. (eds) *Exploring Developmental Psychology from Infancy to Adolescence*. London: Arnold.

Koerner, K. and Dimeff, L. (2000). Further data on dialectical behaviour therapy. *Clinical Psychology Science and Practice*, (7), 104–12.

Kolko, K. and Brent, D. (1988). Cognitive behavioural interventions for adolescent suicide attempters: procedures, processes and preliminary outcomes. Paper presented at the Annual Meeting of the American Psychological Association. Atlanta, August 1988.

Krietman, N. (1977). *Parasuicide*. London: Wiley.

Kreitman, N. (1979). Reflections on the management of parasuicide. *British Journal of Psychiatry*, (135), 275–7.

Kreitman, N. and Casey, P. (1988). Repetition of parasuicide: an epidemiological and clinical study. *British Journal of Psychiatry*, (153), 792–800.

Kroll, L., Woodham, A., Rothwell, J., Bailey, S., Tobias, C., Harrington, R. and Marshal, M. (1999). Reliability of the Salford needs assessment schedule for adolescents. *Psychological Medicine*, (29), 891–902.

Kumar, C., Mohan, R. and Ranjith, G. (2006). Characteristics of high intent suicide attempters admitted to a general hospital. *Journal of Affective Disorders*, 91(1), 77–81.

Lambert, M. and Barley, D. (2001). Research summary on the therapeutic relationship and psychotherapy outcome. *Psychotherapy*, 38(4), 357–61.

Lansdown, G. (2000). Implementing children's rights and health. *Archives of Disease in Childhood*, (83), 286–8.

Lawson, L. and Chaffin, M. (1992). False negatives in sexual abuse disclosure interviews. *Journal of Interpersonal Violence*, 7, 532–42.

Le Surf, A. and Lynch, G. (1999). Exploring young people's perceptions relevant to counselling: a qualitative study. *British Journal of Guidance and Counselling*, 27(2), 231–43.

Lefevre, S. (1996). *Killing Me Softly: self harm – survival not suicide*. Gloucester: Handsell.

Leighton, S. (2006). Nursing children and young people with emotional disorders. In McDougall, T. (ed) *Child and Adolescent Mental Health Nursing*. London: Blackwell.

Leighton, S. (2007). Ethical issues in working therapeutically with vulnerable children. In Vostanis, P. (ed) *Mental Health Interventions and Services for Vulnerable Children and Young People*. London: Jessica Kingsley Publishers.

Lenhart, A., Rainie, L. and Lewis, O. (2001). *Teenage life on–line: the rise of the instant message generation and the Internet's impact on friendships and family relationships*. Washington, DC: Pew Internet and American Life Project.

Letham, J. (1994). *Moved to Tears: moved to Action: brief therapy with women and children*. London: BT Press.

Lewer, L. (2006). Nursing children and young people with eating disorders. In McDougall, T. (ed) *Child and Adolescent Mental Health Nursing*. London: Blackwell.

Lewinsohn, P., Rohde, P. and Seeley, J. (1994). Psychosocial risk factors for future adolescent suicide attempts. *Journal of Consulting and Clinical Psychology*, (62), 297–305.

Lewinsohn, P., Rohde, P. and Seeley, J. (1996). Adolescent suicidal ideation and attempts: prevalence, risk factors and clinical implications. *Clinical Psychology Science and Practice*, (3), 25–46.

Lewisohn, P., Rohde, P. and Seeley, J. (1997). Axis II psychopathology as a function of Axis I disorders in childhood and adolescence. *Journal of the American Academy of Child and Adolescent Psychiatry*, (36), 1752–9.

Liberman, R. and Eckman, T. (1981). Behaviour therapy versus insight orientated therapy for repeated suicide attempters. *Archives of General Psychiatry*, (28), 1126–30.

LifeSigns (2002). LifeSigns Fact Sheet: male self injury. Available at www.lifesigns.org.uk.

Linehan, M. (1993a). *Cognitive Behavioral Therapy of Borderline Personality Disorder*. New York: Guilford.

Linehan, M. (1993b). *Skills Training Manual for Treating Borderline Personality Disorder*. New York: Guilford.

Linehan, M., Armstrong, H., Suarez, A., Allmon, D. and Heard, H. (1991). Cognitive behavioural treatment of chronically parasuicidal borderline patients. *Archives of General Psychiatry*, (48), 1060–4.

Linehan, M., Schmidt, H., Dimeff, L., Craft, J., Kanter, J., Comtois, K. and Recknor, K. (1999). Dialectical behaviour therapy for patients with borderline personality disorder and drug dependence. *American Journal on Addictions*, (8), 279–92.

Livesey, A. (2009). Self harm in adolescent inpatients. *Psychiatric Bulletin*, 33, 10–12.

Low, G., Jones, D., MacLeod, A., Power, M. and Duggan, C. (2000). Childhood trauma, dissociation and self harming behaviour: a pilot study. *British Journal of Medical Psychology*, 73, 269–78.

Lyon, J. (1997). Teenage suicide and self harm: assessing and managing risk. In Kemshall, H. and Pritchard, J. (eds) *Good Practice in Risk Assessment and Management 2: protection, rights and responsibilities*. London: Jessica Kingsley Publishers.

MacAniff, Z. and Kiselica, M. (2001). Understanding and counselling self mutilation in female adolescents and young adults. *Journal of Counselling and Development*, 79(1), 46–52.

Macgowan, M. (2004). Psychosocial treatment of youth suicide: a systematic review of the research. *Research in Social Work Practice*, May, 147–62.

MacLachlin, M. and Smyth, C. (2004). *Binge Drinking and Youth Culture: differing perspectives*. Dublin: Liffey Press.

Madge, N. (1996). *Suicidal Behaviour in Children and Young People: highlight number 144*. London: National Children's Bureau.

Madge, N. and Harvey, J. G. (1999). Suicide among the young – the size of the problem. *Journal of Adolescence*, 22, 145–155.

Madge, N., Hewitt, A., Hawton, K., de Wilde, E., Corcoran, P., Fekete, S., van Heeringen, K., De Leo, D. and Ystgaard, M. (2008). Deliberate self harm within an international community sample of young people: comparative findings from the Child and Adolescent Self Harm in Europe (CASE) Study. *Journal of Child Psychology and Psychiatry*, 49(6), 667–77.

Marciano, P. and Kazdin, A. (1994). Self esteem, depression, hopelessness and suicidal intent among psychiatrically disturbed inpatient children. *Journal of Clinical and Child Psychology*, 23, 151–60.

Martunnen, M., Aro, J., Henriksson, M. and Lonnqvist, J. (1991). Mental disorder in adolescent suicide: DSM III:R Axes I and II diagnoses in suicides among 13–19 year olds in Finland. *Archives of General Psychiatry*, 48, 834–9.

Massie, L. (2008). *Right Time, Right Place: learning from the Children's National Service Framework development initiatives for psychological well–being and mental health, 2005–7*. London: HMSO.

Mayer, J., Salovey, P. and Caruso, D. (2008). Emotional intelligence: new ability or eclectic traits? *American Psychologist*, 63(6), 503–17.

McAuliffe, C., Corcoran, P., Keeley, H. S., Arensman, E., Bille–Brahe, U., De Leo, D., Fekete, S., Hawton, K., Hjelmeland, H., Kelleher, M., Kerkhof, A. J. F. M., Lönnqvist, J., Michel, K., Salander Renberg, E., Schmidtke, A., Van Heeringen, K. and Wasserman, D. (2006). Problem solving ability and repetition of deliberate self harm: a multicentre study. *Psychological Medicine*, (36), 45–55.

McClure, G. (1994). Suicide in children and adolescents in England and Wales. *British Journal of Psychiatry*, 165, 510–14.

McDougall, T. and Brophy, M. (2006). Truth Hurts: young people and self harm. *Mental Health Practice*, 9(9), 14–16.

McDougall, T. and Crocker, A. (2001). Referral pathways through a specialist child mental health service: the role of the specialist practitioner. *Mental Health Practice*, 5(1), 15–20.

McDougall, T. and Jones, C. (2007). Dialectical behaviour therapy for young offenders: lessons from the USA, part 2. *Mental Health Practice*, 11(2), 20–1.

McDougall, T., Pugh, K., O'Herlihey, A. and Parker, C. (2009). Young people on adult mental health wards. *Mental Health Practice*, 12(8), 16–21.

McDougall, T., Worrall–Davies, A., Hewson, L., Richardson, G. and Cotgrove, A. (2007). *Tier 4 Child and Adolescent Mental Health Services: inpatient care, day services and alternatives: an overview of Tier 4 CAMHS provision in the UK*. Child and Adolescent Mental Health.

McKay, D., Hatton, D. and McDougall, T. (2006). Substance misuse, young people and nursing. In McDougall, T. (ed) *Child and Adolescent Mental Health Nursing*. London: Blackwell.

McKenna, K. and Green, A. (2002). Relationship formation on the Internet: what's the big attraction? *Journal of Social Issues*, (58), 9–31.

McLaughlin, J., Miller, P. and Warwick, H. (1996). Deliberate self harm in adolescents: hopelessness, depression, problems and problem solving. *Journal of Adolescence*, (19), 523–32.

McLeavey, B., Daley, R., Ludgate, J. and Murray, C. (1994). Interpersonal problem solving skills training in the treatment of self–poisoning patients. *Suicide and Life Threatening Behaviour*, (24), 382–94.

Meltzer, H., Gatward, R., Goodman, R. and Ford, T. (2001). *Children and adolescents who try to harm, hurt or kill themselves*. London: ONS.

Menninger, K. (1938). *Man against Himself*. New York: Harcourt Brace.

Mental Health Foundation (1999). *Bright Futures*. London: Mental Health Foundation.

Mental Health Foundation and Camelot Foundation (2006). *Truth Hurts: report of the National Inquiry into self harm among young people*. London: Mental Health Foundation.

Merrill, J., Milner, G. and Owens, D. (1992). Alcohol and attempted suicide. *British Journal of Addictions*, 87(1), 83–9.

Merry, S., McDowell, H. and Hetrick, S. (2004). *Psychological and/or Educational Interventions for the Prevention of Depression in Children and Adolescents.* Cochrane Database Systematic Review: Cochrane Database.

Miller, A., Rathus, J. and Linehan, M. (2007). *Dialectical Behavior Therapy with Suicidal Adolescents.* New York: Guildford Press.

Miller, D. (1994). *Women Who Hurt Themselves: a book of hope and understanding.* New York: Basic Books.

MIND (2009). *Information Booklet: MIND guide to advocacy.* London: MIND.

Mitchell, P. (2006). Adolescent forensic mental health nursing. In McDougall, T. (ed) *Child and Adolescent Mental Health Nursing.* London: Blackwell.

Moore, S. and Parsons, J. (2000). A research agenda for adolescent risk taking: where do we go from here? *Journal of Adolescence,* 23, 371–6.

Morano, C., Cisler, R. and Lemerond, J. (1993). Risk Factors for Adolescent Suicidal Behaviour: loss, insufficient familial support and hopelessness. *Adolescence,* 28(1), 24–38.

Morgan, S. (2003). *The Sainsbury's Centre for Mental Health. Assessing and Managing Risk: Practitioners Handbook.* Brighton: Pavilion.

Morris, S. (2008). In harm's way. *Special Children,* June/July, (183), 3–5.

Nation, K. (2003). Developmental language disorders. In Skuse, D. (ed) *Child Psychology and Psychiatry: an Introduction,* 71–4.

National Children's Bureau (2008). *Delivering Every Child Matters in Secure Settings.* London: NCB.

National Collaborating Centre for Mental Health (2005). *Depression in Children and Young People: identification and management in primary, community and secondary care. National Clinical Practice Guideline 28.* London: NICE.

National Collaborating Centre for Mental Health (2009). *Borderline Personality Disorder: the NICE guideline on treatment and management. National Clinical Practice Number 78.* London: NCCMH.

National Collaborating Centre for Women's and Children's Health (2009). *When to Suspect Child Maltreatment.* London: NCCWCH.

National Confidential Inquiry (2009). *National Confidential Inquiry into Suicide and Homicide by People with Mental Illness.* Manchester: NCI.

National Institute for Clinical Excellence (2004a). *Self–harm: The short–term physical and psychological management and secondary prevention of self–harm in primary and secondary care. National Clinical Practice Guideline 16.* London: NICE.

National Institute for Clinical Excellence (2004b). *Core Interventions in the Treatment and Management of Anorexia Nervosa, Bulimia Nervosa and Related Eating Disorders. National Clinical Practice Guideline 9.* London: NICE.

National Institute for Health and Clinical Excellence (2008). *Social and Emotional Wellbeing in Primary Education. (NICE Public Health Guidance 12).* London: NICE.

National Institute for Mental Health in England (2009). *The Legal Aspects of the Care and Treatment of Children and Young People with Mental Disorder: a guide for professionals.* London: NIMHE.

Nav, A., Talbot, P., Siever, L., Frankle, W., Lombardo, I., Goodman, M., Huang, Y., Hwang, D., Slifstem, M., Curry, S., Abi–Dargham, A. and Laurell, M. (2005). Brain serotonin transport distribution in subjects with impulsive aggressivity. *American Journal of Psychiatry,* 162 (suppl.), 915–23.

Nayha, S. (1982). Autumn incidence of suicides re–examined: data from Finland by sex, age and occupation. *British Journal of Psychiatry,* (141), 512–17.

Neale, J., Worrell, M. and Randhawa, G. (2005). Reaching out: support for ethnic minorities. *Mental Health Practice*, 9(2), 12–16.

Nehls, N. (1999). Borderline personality disorder: the voice of patients. *Research in Nursing and Health*, (22), 285–93.

Neill, L. (2003). Market forces: listening to what young people want. *YoungMinds Magazine*, (62), 20–2.

NHS Centre for Reviews and Dissemination (1998). *Effective Health Care: deliberate self harm*. York: NHS CRD.

NHS Health Advisory Service (1995). *Together we Stand: the commissioning, role and management of child and adolescent mental health services*. London: HMSO.

NHS Health Development Agency (2002). *Youth Suicide Prevention: evidence briefing*. London: HDA.

NHS Health Development Agency (2004). *Youth Suicide Prevention: evidence briefing*. Dublin: Institute of Public Health in Ireland.

NHS Scotland (2006). *Talking About Self Harm*. Edinburgh: NHS Scotland.

Nock, M. (2009). Why do people hurt themselves? New insights into the nature and functions of self injury. *Current Directions in Psychological Science*, 18(2), 78–93.

Nock, M., Joiner, T., Gordon, K., Lloyd–Richardson, E. and Prinstein, M. (2009). Non suicidal self injury among adolescents: diagnostic correlates and relation to suicide attempts. *Psychiatry Research*, 144(1), 65–72.

Nolan, B., O'Connell, P. and Whelan, C. (2001). *Bust to boom? the Irish experience of growth and inequality*. Dublin: Economic and Social Research Institute/Institute of Public Administration.

Norris, M., Boydell, K. Pinhas, L. and Katzman, D. (2006). Ana and the Internet: a review of pro–anorexia websites. *International Journal of Eating Disorders*, 39, 443–7.

Northern Ireland Association for Mental Health and Sainsbury Centre for Mental Health (2004). *Counting the Cost*. Belfast: NIAMH and SCMH.

Northern Ireland Statistics and Research Agency (2002). *Northern Ireland Census 2001*. Belfast: NISRA.

Nottingham repeat self harm group for young people (2009). Group exercise. March 2009.

NSPCC (2007). *Self Harm: a ChildLine information sheet*. London: NSPCC.

NSPCC (2008a). *ChildLine Casenotes: children talking to ChildLine about bullying*. London NSPCC.

NSPCC (2008b). *Gillick Competency or Fraser Guidelines: an overview*. London: NSPCC.

NSPCC (2009). *Young People who Self Harm: implications for public health practitioners – child protection research briefing*. London: NSPCC.

O'Driscoll, M. and Holden, N. (2002). *Suicidal Behaviour: awareness and good practice guidelines*. Nottinghamshire: Nottingham Healthcare NHS Trust.

O'Dwyer, F., D'Alton, A. and Pearce, J. (1991). Adolescent self harm patients: audit of assessment in an accident and emergency department. *British Medical Journal*, 303, 629–30.

Office for National Statistics (2006). *Children and Adolescents who try to Harm, Hurt or Kill Themselves*. London: ONS.

Oldershaw, A., Richards, C., Simic, M. and Schmidt, U. (2008). Parent's perspectives on adolescent self–harm: qualitative study. *British Journal of Psychiatry*, (193), 140–4.

Otto, U. (1972). Suicidal acts by children and adolescents: a follow up study. *Acta Psychiatrica Scandinavica*, 233 (suppl.).

Ougrin, D., Ng, A. and Zundel, T. (2009). *Self Harm in Young People: a therapeutic assessment manual*. London: Hodder.

Owens, D., Horrocks, J. and House, A. (2002). Fatal and non fatal repetition of self harm. *British Journal of Psychiatry*, (181), 193–9.

Palmer, L. Blackwell, M. and Stevens, P. (2007). *Service User's Experiences of Emergency Services Following Self Harm: a national survey of 509 patients.* London: College Centre for Quality Improvement: Royal College of Psychiatrists.

Pao, P. (1969). The syndrome of delicate self cutting. *British Journal of Medical Psychology,* 42, 195–206.

PAPYRUS (2008). *Action for Safety on the Internet: the prevention of young suicide.* Burnley: PAPYRUS.

Partonen, T., Haukka, J., Nevanlinna, H. and Lonnqvist, J. (2004). Analysis of the seasonal pattern in suicide. *Journal of Affective Disorders,* 81(2), 133–9.

Pattison, C. and Kahan, J. (1983). The deliberate self harm syndrome. *American Journal of Psychiatry,* (140), 867–72.

Payne, H. and Butler, I. (2003). Promoting the Mental Health of Children in Need. *Research in Practice.* January.

Pembroke, L. (1994). *Self Harm: survivors speak out.* London: Survivors Speak Out.

Perry, S., Cooper, A. and Michels, R. (1987). The psychodynamic formulation. *American Journal of Psychiatry,* 144, 543–50.

Perseius, K., Ojehagen, A. and Ekdahl, S. (2003). Treatment of suicidal and deliberate self–harming patients with borderline personality disorder using dialectical behavioral therapy: the patients' and the therapists' perceptions. *Archives of Psychiatric Nursing,* (17), 218–27.

Pfeffer, C., Klerman, G., Hunt, S., Lesser, M., Peskin, J. and Siefker, A. (1991). Suicidal children grown up: demographic and clinical risk factors for adolescent suicide attempts. *Journal of the American Academy of Child and Adolescent Psychiatry,* (30), 609–16.

Pfeffer, C., Klerman, G., Hurt, S., Kakurma, T., Peskin, J. and Siefker, C. (1993). Suicidal children grown up: rates and psychological risk factors for attempts during follow–up. *Journal of American Academy of Child and Adolescent Psychiatry,* (32), 106–13.

Phillips, D. (1974). The influence of suggestions on suicide: substantive and theoretical implications of the Werther Effect. *American Sociological Review,* (39), 340–54.

Phillips, D. (1982). The impact of fictional television stories on US adult fatalities: new evidence on the effect of the mass media on violence. *American Journal of Sociology,* (87), 1340–59.

Pierce, D. (1997). Suicidal intent in self injury. *British Journal of Psychiatry,* (130), 377–85.

Plant, M. and Plant, M. (1992). *Risk Takers: alcohol, drugs, sex and youth.* London: Routledge.

Platt, S., Bille–Brahe, U., Kerkhoff, J., Schmidtke, A., Bjerke, T., Crepet, P., De Leo, D., Haring, C., Lonnqvist, J. and Michel, K. (1992). Parasuicide in Europe: the WHO/EURO multi centre study on parasuicide 1. Introduction and preliminary analysis for 1989. *Acta Psychiatrica Scandinavica,* 85(2) 97–104.

Ploeg, J., Ciliska, D. and Dobbins, M. (1996). A systematic overview of adolescent suicide prevention programs. *Canadian Journal of Public Health,* (87), 319–24.

Press Complaints Commission Code of Practice. Clause 5. London: PCC.

Princes Trust (2009). *The Princes Trust YouGov Youth Index.* London: Princes Trust.

Pritchard, C. (1995). *Suicide –The Ultimate Rejection? A psychosocial study.* Buckingham: Open University Press.

Pryjmachuk, S. and Trainor, G. (forthcoming 2010). Helping young people who self–harm: perspectives from England. *Journal of Child and Adolescent Psychiatric Nursing,* 23(2).

Public Health Institute of Scotland (2003). *Scottish Needs Assessment report on Child and Adolescent Mental Health.* Glasgow: PHIS.

Pugh, K., McHugh, A. and McKinstrie, F. (2006). *Two steps forward, one step back? 16–25 year olds on their journey to adulthood.* London: YoungMinds.

Raby, C. and Raby, S. (2008). Risk and resilience in childhood. In Jackson, C., Hill, K. and Lavis, P. (eds) *Child and Adolescent Mental Health Today: a handbook*. London: Mental Health Foundation/Pavilion/YoungMinds.

Raleigh, V. and Balajaran, R. (1992). Suicide and self burning among Indians and West Indians in England and Wales. *British Journal of Psychiatry*, 129, 365–8.

Raphael, H., Clarke, G. and Kumar, S. (2006). Exploring parent's responses to their child's deliberate self harm. *Health Education*, 106(1), 9–20.

Rettestol, N. (1993). Death due to overdose of antidepressants: experiences from Norway. *Acta Psychiatrica Scandinavica Supplementum*, (371), 28–32.

Reynolds, W. and Mazza, J. (1993). *Evaluation of suicidal behaviour in adolescents. Reliability of the suicidal behaviour interview*. Unpublished manuscript.

Rhodes, J. and Ajmal, Y. (2004). *Solution Focused Thinking in Schools: behaviour, reading and organisation*. London: BT Press.

Rodham, K., Brewer, H., Mistral, W. and Stallard, P. (2006). Adolescent perceptions of risk and challenge: a qualitative study. *Journal of Adolescence*, (29), 261–72.

Rohde, P. (2005). Cognitive–behavioral treatment for depression in adolescents. *Journal of Indian Child and Adolescent Mental Health* [online journal], 1(1). Available at http://www.jiacam.org/0101/jiacam05_1_6.pdf. Accessed March 2009.

Romans, S., Martin, J., Anderson, J., Herbison, G. and Mullen, P. (1995). Sexual abuse in childhood and deliberate self harm. *American Journal of Psychiatry*, (152), 1336–42.

Rosen, P. and Walsh, B. (1989). Patterns of contagion in self mutilation epidemics. *American Journal of Psychiatry*, (146), 656–8.

Ross, S. and Heath, N. (2002). A study of the frequency of self mutilation in a community sample of adolescents. *Journal of Youth and Adolescence*, 31(1), 67–77.

Rossow, I., Hawton, K. and Ystgaard, M. (2009). Cannabis use and deliberate self harm in adolescence: a comparative analysis of associations in England and Norway. *Archives of Suicide Research*, (13), 340–8.

Rossow, I., Ystgaard, M., Hawton, K., Madge, N., Van Heeringen, K., de Wilde, E. J., De Leo, D., Fekete, S. and Sullivan, C. (2007). Cross national comparisons of the association between alcohol consumption and deliberate self harm in adolescents. *Suicide and Life Threatening Behavior*, (37), 605–15.

Royal College of Paediatrics and Child Health (2003). *Bridging the Gaps: health care for adolescents. Report number CR114*. London: RCPCH.

Royal College of Psychiatrists (1998). *Managing Deliberate Self Harm in Young People. CR64*. London: RCP.

Royal College of Psychiatrists (2004a). *Mental Health and Growing Up. Fact Sheet 17: domestic violence: its effects on children*. London: RCP.

Royal College of Psychiatrists (2004b). *Assessment Following Self Harm in Adults. Council Report CR122*. London: Royal College of Psychiatrists.

Royal College of Psychiatrists (2006). *Better Services for People who Self Harm: quality standards for healthcare professionals*. London: College Research and Training Unit (CRTU).

Ryan, N. (2005). Treatment of depression in children and adolescents. *Lancet*, (366), 933–40.

Ryan, N. and McDougall, T. (2008). *Nursing Children and Young People with ADHD*. London: Routledge.

Sakinofsky, I. (2000). Repetition of suicidal behaviour. In Hawton, K. and van Heeringen, K. (eds) *International Handbook of Suicide and Attempted Suicide*. Chichester: Wiley.

Salkovskis, P., Atha, C. and Storer, D. (1990). Cognitive behaviour problem solving in the treatment of patients who repeatedly attempt suicide: a controlled trial. *British Journal of Psychiatry*, (157), 871–6.

Samaritans (2008). *Media guidelines for reporting suicide and self–harm.* London: Samaritans.

SANE (2007). *Self Harm.* London: SANE.

SANE (2008). Understanding self harm report, by Horne, O. and Paul, S. Available at http://www.sane.org.uk/files/PDF/Research/Understandingself harm.pdf.

Sankey, M. and Lawrence, R. (2005). Brief Report: classification of adolescent suicide and risk–taking deaths. *Journal of Adolescence,* (28), 781–5.

Sansone, R. and Levitt, J. (2002). Self harm behaviors among those with eating disorders: an overview. *Eating Disorders: The Journal of Treatment and Prevention,* 10(3), 205–13.

Santa Mina, E. and Gallop, R. (1998). Childhood sexual and physical abuse and adult self harm and suicidal behaviour: a literature review. *Canadian Journal of Psychiatry,* (43), 793–800.

Saunders, L. and Broad, B. (1997). *The Health Needs of Young People Leaving Care.* Leicester: Leicester University Press.

Scheidinger, S. and Aronson, S. (1991). Group psychotherapy of adolescents. In Slommowitz, M. (ed) *Adolescent psychotherapy: clinical practice.* Washington, DC: American Psychiatric Press.

Schmidtke, A., Bille–Brahe, U., Deleo, D., Kerkhof, A., Bjerke, T., Crepet, P., Haring, C., Hawton, K., Lonnqvist, J., Michel, K., Pommerau, X., Querejeta, I., Phillipe, I., Salander–Renberg, E., Temesvary, B., Wasserman, D., Fricke, S., Weinacker, B. and Sampaio–Faria, J. (1996). Attempted suicide in Europe: rates, trends and socio–demographic characteristics of suicide attempters during the period 1989–92. Results of the WHO/EURO Multicentre Study on Parasuicide. *Acta Psychiatrica Scandinavica,* (93), 327–38.

Schotte, C. and Clum, G. (1987). Problem solving skills in suicidal psychiatric patients. *Journal of Consulting and Clinical Psychology,* 55(1), 49–54.

Schreidman, E. (1993). *Suicide as Psychache.* New York: Wiley.

Scottish Development Centre for Mental Health and the Camelot Foundation (2005). *Building the Strengths Within: improving support for young people from black and ethnic minority groups and communities who self harm or are at risk of self harm.* Edinburgh: SDC.

Scottish Executive (2002a). *Choose Life: a national strategy and action plan to prevent suicide in Scotland.* Edinburgh: Scottish Executive.

Scottish Executive (2002b). *Its Everyone's Job to Make Sure I'm Alright: report of the child protection and audit review.* Edinburgh: The Stationery Office.

Scottish Executive (2008). *Effectiveness of Interventions to Prevent Suicide and Suicidal Behaviour: a systematic review.* Edinburgh: Scottish Government Social Research.

Seinfeld, J. (1996). *Containing Rage, Terror and Despair: an object relations approach to psychotherapy.* London: Aronson.

Sellen, J. (2008). Attitudes matter: working with children and young people who self harm. In Jackson, C., Hill, K. and Lavis, P. (eds) *Child and Adolescent Mental Health Today: a handbook.* London: Pavilion.

Senior, R. (2003). Family and Group Therapies. In Skuse, D. (ed) *Child Psychology and Psychiatry: an introduction,* 165–8.

Shaffer, D. (1974). Suicide in childhood and early ádolescence. *Journal of Child Psychology and Psychiatry,* (15), 275–91.

Shaffer, D., Gould, M. and Brasic, J. (1983). Children's Global Assessment Scale (CGAS). *Archives of General Psychiatry,* (40), 1228–31.

Sharland, E., Seal, H. and Croucher, M. (1996). *Professional Intervention in Child Sexual Abuse.* London: HMSO.

Sheldrick, C. (1999). Practitioner review: the assessment and management of risk in adolescents. *Journal of Child Psychology and Psychiatry,* (40), 507–18.

Simeon, D. and Favazza, A. (2007). Self injurious behaviours, phenomenology and assessment. In Simeon, D. and Hollander, E. (eds) *Self Injurious Behaviours: assessment and treatment*. Washington, DC: American Psychiatric Association.

Sinclair, J. M. A., Gray, A. and Hawton, K. (2006). Systematic review of resource utilization in the short term management of deliberate self harm. *Psychological Medicine*, (36), 1681–94.

Sinclair, J. and Green J. (2005). Understanding resolution of deliberate self harm: qualitative interview study of patient's experiences. *British Medical Journal*, 330, 1112–16.

Singh, S. (2009). *Transition from CAMHS to Adult Mental Health Services (TRACK): a study of service organisation, policies, process and user and carer perspectives: executive summary for the National Coordinating Centre for NHS Service Delivery and Organisation R&D (NCCSDO)*. London: HMSO.

Singleton, N., Meltzer, H. and Gatward, R. (1998). *Psychiatric Morbidity of Prisoners in England and Wales*. London: TSO.

Skegg, K. (2005). Self harm. *The Lancet*, 366(9495), 1471–83.

Smallridge, P. and Williamson, A. (2008). *Independent Review of Restraint in Juvenile Secure Settings*. London: HMSO.

Smith, G., Cox, D. and Saradjian, J. (1998). *Women and self harm*. London: Women's Press.

Smith, K. and Leon, L. (2001). *Turned Upside Down: developing community based crisis services for 16–25 year olds experiencing a mental health crisis*. London: Mental Health Foundation.

Smith, S. (2002). Perceptions of service provision for clients who self–injure in the absence of expressed suicidal intent. *Journal of Psychiatric and Mental Health Nursing*, 9(5), 595–601.

Social Care Institute for Excellence (2005). *SCIE Research Briefing 16: deliberate self harm (DSH) among children and adolescents: who is at risk and how is it recognised?* London: SCIE.

Spandler, H. (1996). *Who's hurting who? young people, self harm and suicide*. Manchester: 42nd St.

Spandler, H. (2001). *Who's hurting who? young people, self harm and suicide*. (2nd edition). Gloucester: Handsell.

Spandler, H. and Warner, S. (2007). *Beyond Fear and Self Control: working with young people who self harm*. Ross–on–Wye: PCSS Books.

Speckens, A. and Hawton, K. (2005). Social problem solving in adolescents with suicidal behaviour: a systematic review. *Suicide and Life Threatening Behavior*, (35), 365–87.

Spirito, A., Brown, L., Overholser, J. and Fritz, G. (1989). Attempted suicide in adolescence: a review and critique of the literature. *Clinical Psychology Review*, (9), 335–63.

Stanard, R. (2000). Assessment and treatment of adolescent depression and suicidality. *Journal of Mental Health Counselling*, 22(3), 204–17.

Stirn, A. and Hinz, A. (2008). Tattoos, body piercings and self injury: is there a connection? Investigations on a core group of participants practicing body modification. *Psychotherapy Research*, 18(3), 326–33.

Subrahmanyam, K., Greenfield, P. and Tynes, B. (2004). Constructing sexuality and identity in an online teen chat room. *Journal of Applied Developmental Psychology*, (25), 651–66.

Suyemoto, K. (1998). The functions of self–mutilation. *Clinical Psychology Review*, 18(5), 531–554.

Tameside Children and Young People Strategic Partnership. *Parent Power: a strategy for supporting and involving parents in Tameside*. Tameside: Tameside Metropolitan Borough Council.

Taylor, S., Rider, I., Turkington, D., MacKenzie, J. and Garside, M. (2006). Does a specialist team impact on repetition rates and discharge outcomes following the first episode of self harm? *Mental Health Practice*, 9(7), 30–2.

Taylor, T. L., Hawton, K., Fortune, S. and Kapur, N. (2009). Attitudes towards clinical services among people who self harm: systematic review. *British Journal of Psychiatry*, (194), 104–10.

Thomas–Boyce, W. and Ellis, B. (2005). Biological sensitivity to context: an evolutionary–developmental theory of the origins and function of stress reactivity. *Developmental Psychopathology*, 17, 271–301.

Thomas, P., Schroeter, K., Dahmee, B. and Nutzinger, D. (2002). Self injurious behaviour in women with eating disorders. *American Journal of Psychiatry*, 159, 408–11.

Thompson, E., Eggert, L. and Herting, J. (2000). Mediating effects of an indicated prevention programme for reducing youth depression and suicide risk behaviours. *Suicide and Life Threatening Behaviour*, (30), 252–71.

Timimi, S. (2007). Should young people be given antidepressants? No. *British Medical Journal*, 335, 750.

Torhorst, A., Moller, H., Burk, F., Kurz, A., Wachtler, C. and Lauter, H. (1987). The psychiatric management of parasuicide patients: a controlled clinical study comparing different strategies for outpatient treatment. *Crisis*, (8), 53–61.

Townsend, E., Hawton, K., Altman, D., Arensman, E., Gunnell, D., Hazell. P., House, A. and van Heeringen, K. (2001). The efficacy of problem solving treatments after deliberate self harm: meta–analysis of randomised controlled trials with respect to depression, hopelessness and improvement in problems. *Psychological Medicine*, 31(6), 979–88.

Turvill, J., Burroughs, A. and Moore, K. (2000). Change in occurrence of paracetamol overdose in UK after introduction of blister packs. *Lancet*, (355), 2048–9.

UNICEF (2007). *An Overview of Child Wellbeing in Rich Countries: a comprehensive assessment of the lives and well–being of children and adolescents in the economically advanced nations.* UNICEF: Florence.

United States Department of Health and Human Services (1981). *Health: United States DHSS.* Myatsville, Maryland.

Utting, W. (1997). *People like Us: the report of the review of safeguards for children living away from home.* London: TSO.

Vajda, J. and Steinbeck, K. (1999). Factors associated with repeat suicide attempts among adolescents. *Australian and New Zealand Journal of Psychiatry*, (34), 437–45.

van der Sande, R., van Rooijen, E., Buskens, E., Allart, E., Hawton, K. and van der Graaf, Y. (1997). Intensive patient and community intervention versus routine care after attempted suicide: a randomised controlled trial. *British Journal of Psychiatry*, (171), 35–41.

van Heeringen, C., Jannes, S., Buylaert, H., Hendrick, H., de Banquer, D. and van Remoortel, J. (1995). The management of non compliance with referral to outpatient after care among attempted suicide patients: a controlled intervention study. *Psychological Medicine*, (25), 963–70.

Walsh, B. (2006). *Treating Self Injury: a practical guide.* New York: Guilford Press.

Walsh, B. and Rosen, P. (1988). *Self Mutilation: theory, research and treatment.* New York: Guilford.

Waterhouse, J. and Platt, S. (1990). General hospital admission in the management of parasuicide. *British Journal of Psychiatry*, (156), 236–42.

Webb, L. (2002). Deliberate self–harm in adolescence: a systematic review of psychological and psychosocial factors. *Journal of Advanced Nursing*, 38 (3), 235–44.

Weinberg, I., Gunderson, J. and Hennen, J. (2006). Manual assisted cognitive treatment for deliberate self harm in borderline personality disorder patients. *Journal of Personality Disorders*, (20), 482–92.

Wells, J., Barlow, J. and Stewart–Brown, S. (2003). A systematic review of universal approaches to mental health promotion in schools. *Health Education*, 103, 197–220.

Welsh Assembly Government (2008). *Talk to Me: a national action plan to reduce suicide and self harm in Wales 2008–13.* Cardiff: Welsh Assembly Government.

Welsh Office (1997). *The Health of Children in Wales.* Cardiff: Welsh Office.

Welu, T. (1977). A follow up programme for suicide attempters: evaluation of effectiveness. *Suicide and Life Threatening Behaviour*, (7), 17–30.

Whitlock, J., Powers, J. and Eckenrode, J. (2006). The virtual cutting edge: the Internet and adolescent self injury. *Developmental Psychology*, 42(3), 1–11.

Whittington, C., Kendall, T., Fonagy, P., Cottrell, D., Cotgrove, A. and Boddington, E. (2004). Selective serotonin reuptake inhibitors in childhood depression: systematic review of published versus unpublished data. *Lancet*, 363, 1341–5.

Whotton, E. (2002). What to do when an adolescent self harms. *Emergency Nurse*, 10(5), 12–16.

Williams, R. (2008). Resilience and risk in children and young people. In Jackson, C., Hill, K. and Lavis, P. (eds) *Child and Adolescent Mental Health Today: a handbook*. London: Mental Health Foundation/Pavilion/YoungMinds.

Winchel, R. and Stanley, M. (1991). Self injurious behaviour: a review of the behaviour and biology of self mutilation. *American Journal of Psychiatry*, (148), 306–17.

Windfhur, K. (2008). Suicides in juveniles and adolescents in the United Kingdon. *Journal of Child Psychology and Psychiatry*, (49), 1155–65.

Windfhur, K. (2009). Issues in designing, implementing and evaluating suicide prevention strategies. *Psychiatry*, 8(7), 272–5.

Winnicott, D. W. (1965) [2001]. *The Family and Individual Development*. East Sussex: Brunner–Routledge.

Wolpert, M., Fuggle, P., Cottrell, D., Fonagy, P., Phillips, J., Pilling, S., Stein, S. and Target, M. (2006). *Drawing on the Evidence: advice for mental health professionals working with children and adolescents*. London: CAMHS Publications.

Wood, A. J., Harrington, R. C., Moore, A. (1996). Controlled trial of a brief cognitive behavioural intervention in adolescent patients with depressive disorders. *Journal of Child Psychology and Psychiatry*, 37, 737–46.

Wood, A., Trainor, G., Rothwell, J., Moore, A. and Harrington, R. (2001). A randomized controlled trial of group therapy for repeated deliberate self–harm in adolescents. *Journal of the American Academy of Child and Adolescent Psychiatry*, (40), 1246–53.

Woodroffe, C., Glickman, M., Barker, M. and Power, C. (1993). *Young Persons, Teenagers and Health: key data*. Buckingham: Open University Press.

Woolley, I. (2006). Treatment interventions for children and young people with mental health problems. In McDougall, T. (ed) *Child and Adolescent Mental Health Nursing*. London: Blackwell Publishing.

World Health Organization (1993). *The ICD–10 Classification of Mental and Behavioural Disorders: clinical descriptions and diagnostic guidelines*. Geneva: WHO.

World Health Organization (1997). *Child Mental Health and Psychosocial Development: technical report series 613*. Geneva: WHO.

World Health Organization (2000a). *Preventing Suicide: a resource for media professionals*. Geneva: WHO.

World Health Organization (2000b). *Preventing Suicide: a resource for health care professionals*. Geneva: WHO.

World Health Organization (2009). *European Health for All Database (HFA–DB)*. Geneva: WHO.

Worrall, A., Boylan, J. and Roberts, D. (2008). *Children's and Young People's Experiences of Domestic Violence Involving Adults in a Parenting Role*. London: Social Care Institute for Excellence.

Wright, B. and Richardson, G. (2003). In Richardson, G. and Partridge, I. (eds) *Child and Adolescent Mental Health Services: an operational handbook*. London: Gaskell.

Yates, T. (2004). The developmental psychopathology of self injurious behavior: compensatory regulation in posttraumatic adaptation. *Clinical Psychological Review*, (24), 35–74.

Yip, P. S. F., Fu, K. W., Yang, K. C. T., Ip, B. Y. T., Chan, C. L. W., Chen, E. Y. H., Less, D. T. S., Law, F. Y. W. and Hawton, K. (2006). The effects of a celebrity suicide on suicide rates in Hong Kong. *Journal of Affective Disorders*, (93), 245–52.

Young, D. and Gunderson, J. (1995). Family images of borderline adolescents. *Psychiatry*, 58, 164–72.

Young, R., Sweeting, H. and West, P. (2006). Prevalence of deliberate self harm and attempted suicide within contemporary Goth youth subculture: longitudinal cohort study. *British Medical Journal*, 332, 1058–61.

Young, R., van Beinum, M., Sweeting, H. and West, P. (2007). Young people who self harm. *British Journal of Psychiatry*, 191, 44–9.

YoungMinds (1999). *Mental Health in Children and Young People: spotlight (No. 1 in a series of briefing papers)*. London: YoungMinds.

YoungMinds (2006). *See Beyond the Label: empowering young people who self harm: a training manual*. London: YoungMinds.

YoungMinds (2008). *See Beyond the Label*. London: YoungMinds.

YoungMinds (2009). *Poll reveals young people are still not getting support: press release*. London: YoungMinds.

Youth Justice Board (2006). *Health Needs Assessment for Young Women in Young Offender Institutions*. London: YJB.

Ystgaard, M., Arensman, E., Hawton, K., Madge, N., Van Heeringen, K., Hewitt, A., de Wilde, E. J., De Leo, D. and Fekete, S. (2009). Deliberate self harm in adolescents: comparison between those who receive help following self harm and those who do not. *Journal of Adolescence*, (32), 875–91.

Zahl, D. and Hawton, K. (2004). Repetition of deliberate self harm and subsequent follow up study in 11,583 patients. *British Journal of Psychiatry*, 185, 70–5.

Zigmund, A. and Snaith, R. (1983). The Hospital Anxiety and Depression Rating Scale. *Acta Scandinavica Psychiactrica*, (67), 361–70.

Zimmerman,T., Jacobson, R., MacIntyre, Y. and Watson, C. (1996). Solution Focused Parenting Groups: an empirical study. *Journal of Family Therapy*, 19, 159–72.

Online resources

The following links take readers to useful resources:

42nd Street
www.fortysecondstreet.org.uk

The Basement Project
www.basementproject.co.uk

Better Services for People who Self Harm
www.rcpsych.ac.uk/crtu/
centreforqualityimprovement/servicesforself–
harm.aspx

Bristol Crisis Services for Women
www.selfinjurysupport.org.uk

LifeLink
www.lifelink.org.uk

LifeSigns
www.lifesigns.org.uk

Mental Health Foundation
www.mentalhealth.org.uk

National Self Harm Network
www.nshn.co.uk

Newham Asian Women's Project
www.nawp.org

Oxford Centre for Suicide Research
http://cebmh.warne.ox.ac.uk/csr

Papyrus
www.papyrus–uk.org

Parent Line Plus
www.parentlineplus.org.uk

Penumbra
www.penumbra.org.uk

Samaritans
www.samaritans.org

Self Harm Alliance
www.selfharmalliance.org

Self Harm Recovery, Advice and Support
www.thesite.org/healthandwellbeing/
mentalhealth/selfharm

TheSite
www.thesite.org

YoungMinds
www.youngminds.org.uk

Index

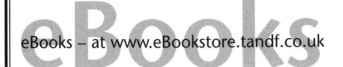